Dementia: A Very Short Introduction

VERY SHORT INTRODUCTIONS are for anyone wanting a stimulating and accessible way into a new subject. They are written by experts, and have been translated into more than 45 different languages.

The series began in 1995, and now covers a wide variety of topics in every discipline. The VSI library currently contains over 650 volumes—a Very Short Introduction to everything from Psychology and Philosophy of Science to American History and Relativity—and continues to grow in every subject area.

Very Short Introductions available now:

Available soon:

For more information visit our website

www.oup.com/vsi/

Kathleen Taylor

DEMENTIA

A Very Short Introduction

OXFORD
UNIVERSITY PRESS

Great Clarendon Street, Oxford, OX2 6DP,
United Kingdom

Oxford University Press is a department of the University of Oxford.
It furthers the University's objective of excellence in research, scholarship,
and education by publishing worldwide. Oxford is a registered trade mark of
Oxford University Press in the UK and in certain other countries

Published in the United States of America by Oxford University Press
198 Madison Avenue, New York, NY 10016, United States of America

British Library Cataloguing in Publication Data
Data available

Library of Congress Control Number: 2020932448

ISBN 978-0-19-882578-4

Printed in Great Britain by
Ashford Colour Press Ltd, Gosport, Hampshire

Contents

List of illustrations

Abbreviations

ACh	acetylcholine
AD	Alzheimer's disease
ADI	Alzheimer's Disease International
ALS	amyotrophic lateral sclerosis
APOE	apolipoprotein E
APP	amyloid precursor protein
BACE	beta-secretase (beta-site amyloid precursor protein cleaving enzyme)
BSE	bovine spongiform encephalopathy
CBT	cognitive behavioural therapy
CJD	Creutzfeldt-Jakob disease
COPD	chronic obstructive pulmonary disease
CSF	cerebrospinal fluid
CT	computer tomography
DLB	Dementia with Lewy bodies
DNA	deoxyribonucleic acid
DSM	*Diagnostic and Statistical Manual*
EEG	electroencephalography
fMRI	functional MRI
FTD	frontotemporal dementia
GABA	gamma-aminobutyric acid
GBD	global burden of disease
HDL	high-density lipoprotein
HIV	human immunodeficiency virus

ICD	*International Classification of Diseases*
LATE	limbic-predominant age-related TDP-43 encephalopathy
LDL	low-density lipoprotein
MCI	mild cognitive impairment
MEG	magnetoencephalography
MRI	magnetic resonance imaging
NCD	neurocognitive disorder
NHD	Nasu-Hakola disease
NIH	National Institutes of Health
NPIs	non-pharmacological interventions
PET	positron emission tomography
PLOSL	polycystic lipomembranous osteodysplasia with sclerosing leukoencephalopathy
PSEN	presenilin
RCT	randomized controlled trial
RNA	ribonucleic acid
TBI	traumatic brain injury
TREM2	triggering receptor expressed on myeloid 2
UV	ultraviolet radiation
vCJD	variant Creutzfeldt-Jakob disease
WHO	World Health Organization

Chapter 1
The challenges of dementia

Brain illnesses are one of the toughest challenges we humans face. They have a huge impact on length and quality of life, and they take many forms: neurodevelopmental disorders like epilepsy and autism, mental health problems like depression and anxiety, neurodegenerative conditions like Alzheimer's and Parkinson's diseases. The topic of this book, dementia, is one of the commonest types of brain ill-health, and one of the most feared.

According to Alzheimer's charities, in the UK there are 200,000 new cases per year and over 850,000 people living with the condition. In the USA, it's estimated that 5.8 million people have Alzheimer's, with over 480,000 developing it in 2019. Worldwide, around 50 million people are thought to have it. In England and Wales, dementia is now the number one cause of death. In 2016, the World Health Organization (WHO)'s enormous Global Burden of Disease (GBD) study placed it fifth, with almost two (1.99) million deaths per year. That toll was surpassed only by heart disease (9.43 million), stroke (5.78 million), chronic obstructive pulmonary disease (COPD, one of the world's most under-recognized killers, with 3.04 million), and lower respiratory infections, such as pneumonia (2.96 million). A 2017 update and reanalysis of the GBD data showed that more people now die with dementia than with diabetes, or with lung cancer, or stomach and bowel cancers, or from road accidents.

We think of dementia as a problem of old age. Yet it can occur in younger people, and even, in rare genetic cases, in childhood—with severe impacts on life, work, and family. And though dementia is mostly found in older folk, its negative effects reach far beyond them: to carers, relatives, and anyone who fears for their future. It is a major concern for health and social care services and the taxpayers who fund them. With populations in many countries ageing rapidly, the challenges of dementia are only going to become more urgent.

The concept of dementia began, not as a disease, but as a collection of symptoms affecting an individual's ability to think and function independently. This is still key to how dementia is diagnosed: a person must be impaired in at least two different cognitive domains, and so impaired that it is seriously interfering with their ability to manage their life. Cognitive domains include memory, language, attention, problem-solving, and 'orientation', the capacity to know when, where, and who one is. Such symptoms are part of many brain disorders. They can also occur after severe physical ordeals such as surgery or head injury. They tell us that a brain is struggling to cope with the demands on it. That may be because of short-term, temporary problems such as a failing blood supply, or longer-term, irreversible ones such as loss of brain tissue.

Even when symptoms are temporary, and the person appears to recover from, say, major surgery, they may not get back quite the cognitive capacities they had—especially if they are elderly. They may also go on to experience faster cognitive decline than one would expect in healthy ageing.

When the symptoms are part of a progressive illness, worsening until life is unsustainable, they are thought to be caused by one of the set of terminal brain diseases lumped together as 'dementia'. The most common of these are vascular dementia, frontotemporal dementia, dementia with Lewy bodies, and, most frequent of all,

Alzheimer's. Alzheimer's is the best known and the most studied, and the scientific attempts to understand and treat that form of dementia will be the main focus of this book, though I will also discuss other types (for example in Chapters 4 and 5).

From past to present

For a condition so associated with old age, dementia in the modern medical sense is quite a young concept. It owes its beginnings to the great surge of interest in, and knowledge of, human brains and their workings in the later 19th and early 20th centuries. Researchers and clinicians mapped the human brain, traced out its pathways, and developed many of the foundational techniques of neuroscience, from electrode recordings and lesion studies to cell staining and dissection. (A lesion is a localized area of brain damage, and depending on its location it can cause extraordinary symptoms, such as profound religious experiences, the inability to see movement, or the belief that loved ones have been replaced by impostors. Cell staining uses chemicals which bind to particular components or types of brain cell, 'highlighting' them so they stand out from the mass of surrounding brain tissue.)

Some enlightened doctors also looked for better ways of understanding their patients, and that involved studying and categorizing them. As part of this work, they examined the brains of patients who had died of 'senile dementia', in the hope of finding ways to treat the condition.

Cognitive problems have long been recognized as a threat of advancing age, often with profound consequences for the afflicted individual's place in society. In classical Greece, for example, having what we now call dementia altered a person's legal rights. The word itself is of Latin origin (*demens*, 'from, or out of, the mind'), and the Roman writer Cicero—in his *De Senectute*, 'Of Old Age'—clearly distinguishes between the healthy and unhealthy ageing of mental faculties. However, it took until the first decade of the 20th century to identify specific markers of disease.

The man whose name is forever linked to this achievement was Aloysius ('Alois') Alzheimer, a German neuroscientist and doctor. Using the new cell staining techniques developed by his colleague—and best man—Franz Nissl, Alzheimer detected abnormalities in the brain of a female dementia patient, Auguste Deter. 'Auguste D.', as she became known to science, was admitted to hospital in 1901, and was under Alzheimer's care until she died—five years later and still only in her fifties. Her symptoms included memory loss, confusion, disorientation, and delirium. Research has since shown that the abnormalities Alzheimer identified are much more common in the brains of people with dementia than they are in healthy brains of similar age.

Alzheimer was part of a new wave of scientific attempts to link psychiatric symptoms to brain problems. One of his most influential colleagues was Emil Kraepelin, a founder of modern psychiatry. Kraepelin saw dementia as a separate clinical entity from depression, personality disorders, and the archetypal form of madness, 'dementia praecox' (schizophrenia), with its delusions and hallucinations. It was he who coined the term Alzheimer's. Alois himself referred only to 'an unusual illness of the cerebral cortex'. He seems to have been a modest man as well as a respected and humane clinician.

Ironically, Auguste D. probably didn't have Alzheimer's dementia. Following re-examination of Alzheimer's original data, she is now thought to have had a similar but rarer condition called Pick's disease.

Here is part of Alzheimer's (translated) description of his patient, from his 1901 case notes:

At lunch she eats cauliflower and pork. Asked what she is eating she answers *spinach*. When she was chewing meat and asked what she was doing, she answered *potatoes* and then *horseradish*. When objects are shown to her, she does not remember after a short time which objects have been shown. In between she always speaks about twins. When she is asked to write, she holds the book in such a way that one has the impression that she has a loss in the right visual field. Asked to write Auguste D, she tries to write Mrs and forgets the rest. It is necessary to repeat every word.

. . .

On what street do you live? *I can tell you, I must wait a bit*. What did I ask you? *Well, this is Frankfurt am Main*. On what street do you live? *Waldemarstreet, not, no.* ... When did you marry? *I don't know at present. The woman lives on the same floor*. Which woman? *The woman where we are living*. The patient calls *Mrs G, Mrs G, here a step deeper, she lives.* ... I show her a key, a pencil and a book and she names them correctly. What did I show you? *I don't know, I don't know*. It's difficult isn't it? *So anxious, so anxious*. I show her 3 fingers; how many fingers? *3*. Are you still anxious *Yes*. How many fingers did I show you? *Well this is Frankfurt am Main*.

In Alzheimer's time, dementia was seen as a potentially treatable group of illnesses, subdivided into senile and presenile dementia (Auguste D. had the presenile type). They were considered quite distinct. Presenile dementias were rare diseases, whereas opinion varied as to whether senile dementia was an illness or an inevitable consequence of ageing. In the 1970s, the story changed when researcher Robert Katzman published an article arguing that presenile and senile dementia were the same disease. In doing so, he helped create modern dementia research. Today, scientists and clinicians still distinguish early- and late-onset dementia, with the border usually set at age 60 or 65. But they see both as arising from similar, damaging brain changes, leading to the death of cells, that are collectively known as neurodegeneration.

As Katzman was writing, techniques were being developed which would allow researchers to look inside living brains, digitally record, store, and analyse vast quantities of information, and manipulate genes. Together, these technological advances have transformed our understanding of how human brains work—and fail. Meanwhile, ageing and massively larger populations have concentrated many minds on the issue of how to care for the unwell elderly, making dementia research a national and international priority. As dementia emerges from its long, stigmatized silence, people with the condition are finding their voices, personally and politically, giving us more individual experiences of living with dementia. (A powerful example is the acclaimed 2018 memoir by Wendy Mitchell, *Somebody I Used to Know*.) With the higher profile has come more advocacy: for funding, better care, and for dementia to be considered a disability rather than a fearful and absolute death sentence. Thus for example the Alzheimer Society of Canada has set out a Charter of Rights for people with dementia (it can be found at <https://alzheimer.ca/en/Home/Get-involved/The-Charter>). As more people are diagnosed earlier, and with disability rights in general becoming more of a priority, these trends are likely to continue.

Symptoms

Dementia is usually thought of as a problem with cognition and, especially, memory. Subjective complaints of the 'where did I put my keys?' variety cause a lot of concern as people grow older. They are a predictor of dementia; that is, they are associated with a greater chance of the condition developing. Thus it makes sense for doctors to keep an eye on people alarmed by such lapses—even if they pass the doctor's tests of cognition. Then again, 'a greater chance' is not certainty, nor is prediction doom. Memory complaints do not inevitably signal either incipient dementia or the syndrome known as 'mild cognitive impairment' (MCI), just as MCI does not inevitably lead to dementia. Older brains tend to work a little more slowly, and to use different strategies, than younger ones, and part of this involves prioritizing their resources to pay attention to what they consider important. Often an older person will be well able to remember material that matters to them, even when they can't recall casual everyday details, like where they put the keys.

Besides, memory is an effortful process. It can easily be made worse by chronic stress, fatigue, and anxiety, as well as by ageing. Using recreational or medical drugs can also impact on memory; so can sleep loss and the menopause. Alcohol's short-term effects are well known, but long-term heavy drinking can be ruinous. Having certain medical conditions, including diabetes, depression, and epilepsy, can also affect memory. Other causes need to be ruled out before memory problems can be assigned to MCI or dementia.

Typically, however, dementia appears first as short-term memory failures, word-finding difficulties, and suchlike. It progresses to more troubling difficulties. Talking to others, a person may struggle to follow the conversation, or forget what they were saying, or repeat themselves with no awareness of having done so. (A carer for someone with dementia soon learns not to draw attention to such lapses: it only makes the person more anxious, and their symptoms worse.) Dealing with household management, individuals with dementia may omit to pay bills or forget appointments; they may find their finances unmanageable, and everyday tasks like shopping problematic. I had an elderly relative with vascular dementia, and one of her more bewildering symptoms in the early stages involved buying vast stocks of food—because she would forget what she already had. For a while it was sausages, then bags of chips, then ice-cream. (By that time her son-in-law was already, surreptitiously, dealing with her finances; she had simply given up on paying bills.)

Life's demands, in today's complex and high-tech societies, are extensive. They put a lot of strain on all brains, not just older ones.

This increased cognitive load may have helped to make dementia more visible than before.

As the condition progresses—this medical use of the term 'progress' lacks the usual hopeful overtones—the person may lose all sense of dates and current events. This is why establishing whether someone has dementia often involves asking questions like, 'Who is the Prime Minister?' or, 'What was in the news this morning?' As memory decays, the perception of time can shrink to a narrow window. (For my relative, awareness of the future and the past all but vanished, leaving her with an eternal now that she described as 'drifting'.) Occasional memories can still be triggered, but they become more distant and infrequent. People with dementia may no longer know their age, their name, or where they are and why. They may also lose the capacity to recognize others, even close loved ones. This is one of the most painful and dreaded symptoms.

Not all memory is equally affected, however. Consciously retrieving information typically becomes more difficult, whereas learned skills may be retained. The ability to find words or recognize faces may diminish faster than, say, music recognition. To complicate matters further, there are cases of dementia in which other cognitive domains are affected but memory problems are not a notable symptom.

Even 'typical' dementia, however, is a problem with more than just memory for things, events, and people. One of the earliest symptoms is difficulty with finding one's way around familiar places. Someone may go shopping, only to become disoriented and unable to make their way home. In less familiar places, or if the person is moved from a well-known home to, say, a care home, the symptoms may suddenly worsen. This can be extremely distressing for families trying to do the right thing by their loved one.

The control of attention and alertness may also be affected. The person may drift off, stare into space, or be unable to complete tasks. Sentences may jump from topic to topic, fizzle out uncompleted, or seem unrelated to the flow of conversation. Other cognitive symptoms include failures of reasoning and understanding which can be apparent from talking to the person with dementia. He or she may appear to hold bizarre beliefs—although this, like not knowing the Prime Minister's name, is not exclusive to dementia.

Sometimes the beliefs seem paranoid, or detached from reality, but often one can work out possible reasons for them. On one family visit to my relative, for example, the visitors, who lived nearby, found her convinced they had come over from America to see her. I can only think that this was because I'd visited the week before and mentioned the States: another family member was holidaying there. One of the most disconcerting aspects of dementia is that you never know what will stick in the mind.

Dementia is mainly talked about as a cognitive problem, but it is also an emotional and behavioural one. This is unsurprising, given the disorientation and confusion patients experience; but their ability to regulate and understand their emotions also seems to worsen as the disease progresses. Alzheimer himself was a clear-eyed and compassionate observer of his patient's suffering, noting how she screamed and cried, terrified in a situation which made no sense to her. The nature of the emotional disturbances seems to depend on illness stage, and on the person's situation, care, and perhaps pre-existing personality. Behavioural problems, which can also be very challenging for carers, include aggressive and agitated behaviour, wandering, difficulties with eating and drinking, and incontinence.

In addition, the condition varies greatly from day to day, and even hour to hour. One of the symptoms my family found most disturbing was that our relative would have flashes of lucidity.

They usually lasted just long enough for her to realize that something was very wrong—and panic, to her great distress and ours. Tiredness, low blood sugar, stress, and infections can all worsen symptoms. Indeed, some infections can be accompanied by delirium, and this mental confusion can be mistaken for dementia, especially in elderly patients. Routines, good healthcare, exercise, and nutrition, and being lovingly cared for in a safe and familiar environment, can keep symptoms stable, or at least slow the rate of decline.

Symptoms can also vary with the type of dementia a person has—and which brain regions are most affected. For example, frontotemporal dementia, as the name suggests, particularly affects the frontal lobe, which is involved in many social and regulatory functions, from moral judgement to empathy to the inhibition of inappropriate behaviours. Damage to this part of the brain can transform personality. Sometimes this can be an improvement; my relative's sharp tongue definitely mellowed. In less fortunate cases, a kindly grandmother may become a foul-mouthed bigot, or a gentle husband a violent stranger. Other types of dementia too can show changes, including paranoid or inappropriate behaviour, wandering, emotional volatility, and inability to control one's reactions. Sensory and motor functions can also be affected, leading to confusion, difficulties with everyday tasks, problems maintaining posture, and a greater risk of falls. Dementia with Lewy bodies (DLB), for instance, often involves problems with movement akin to those seen in Parkinson's—such as tremor and disrupted gait—along with sleep disorders, disturbances of vision, and hallucinations.

As dementia progresses, the person typically becomes less mobile, more physically frail, and less able to live independently. They are less likely to initiate a movement or conversation and more likely to give stock responses. As well as memory, speech capacities fall away, though even in advanced dementia the person may still respond to music: emotional responses generally last longer. Physical difficulties, such as with eating, dressing, and toilet functions, increase. There may be significant weight change. Experiencing pain and confusion, the person may be frustrated by their inability to communicate their suffering. One of the major developments of recent years has been in understanding problem behaviours in terms of people trying to communicate, rather than as due to brain malfunction (which denies them agency) or 'acting up' (which misattributes it).

Eventually the person with dementia may become bed-bound, with associated risks such as bedsores, and their physical functions will deteriorate. In the end-stage of dementia, during the last few days of life, there is usually a noticeable speeding-up of the decline, as the body's ability to maintain itself collapses. Many individuals with dementia, however, never reach this stage, as some other illness intervenes.

Dementia in the brain

Dementia is a clinical diagnosis, on the basis of symptoms experienced by a human being. Some causes of dementia are neurodegenerative disorders affecting a human brain; but the match between cause and symptoms is not straightforward. It is possible to have dementia (a set of symptoms) without evidence of neurodegeneration. It is also possible, as we shall see, to have signs of neurodegeneration ('pathology') without the cognitive symptoms of dementia. Take for example Alzheimer's disease. Clinicians may suspect its presence—coding a patient's condition as 'probable Alzheimer's' or 'dementia of the Alzheimer type'—but definitive diagnosis requires the pathological assessment of brain tissue. Traditionally, this has been done by post-mortem analysis, still the 'gold standard' method of confirming or rejecting clinical judgements. Yet a 2019 study of 180 brains found mismatches between the clinical and pathological diagnoses in over a third of cases.

Neurodegeneration involves damage to and death of brain cells, but this can happen in various ways, giving rise to differing rates of progression, differences in which brain regions are affected (and when), and different symptoms. Sometimes the process can be devastatingly swift: Creutzfeldt-Jakob disease (prion disease, CJD) can take a patient from diagnosis to death within a year. Typically, however, neurodegeneration progresses more slowly. Dementia, ataxia, Parkinson's, Huntington's, and motor neuron disease (amyotrophic lateral sclerosis, ALS) may be lived with for years or decades.

To understand neurodegeneration, we need to look at the brain cells it affects. The best known of these are neurons, which transmit electrical signals through the brain. They typically have a stout cell body, enclosed in a fatty membrane, with one long projection known as an axon, and many short ones called dendrites. Axons carry the neuron's signals to synapses (named from the Greek *syn-haptein*, 'to touch together'). These are tiny gaps between a cell and its neighbours; there are many trillions of synapses in a human brain. Dendrites receive incoming signals from other cells. Axons can cover great lengths: more than a metre in humans (the distance from your spinal cord to your toes). Dendrites are much shorter, a few millimetres or less, but far more plentiful.

Neurons communicate using chemicals known as neurotransmitters, molecules released by one cell into the tiny synaptic gap between it and its neighbour. Neurotransmitters float across the gap and form chemical bonds with specialized receptor molecules on the neighbour's membrane. This changes the receptor's shape, triggering complex changes in the receiving cell. The result is to excite—or inhibit—its electrical activity, raising—or lowering—the chance that it too will transmit the message by sending a signal of its own. Most neurons in the cortex use either the excitatory neurotransmitter glutamate or the inhibitory one GABA (gamma-aminobutyric acid).

Scientists think that neurodegeneration usually begins with the loss of synapses, followed by dendrites dying off and axon failure. Eventually the cell itself dies, and when this happens its contents can be released. Many of these are toxic—in a healthy cell they are kept in special internal compartments—and so organisms have evolved efficient clean-up mechanisms for sick and dying cells. Unfortunately, these work less well in older bodies, and as neurodegeneration takes hold they can be overwhelmed. That leads to an ever more poisoned cellular environment, and more cells dying.

Much research into dementia is focused on identifying how neurodegeneration starts, and on stopping it early, or preventing it altogether. That is likely to be an easier prospect than trying to reverse it or clearing up the damage later on.

The anatomy of decline

How does neurodegeneration affect the brain as a whole? To see that, we need to take a look at brain structure. Figure 1 shows a schematic outline of a human brain, seen from the left side. At its base is the brainstem, through which signals flow from brain to spinal cord to body and back again. The brainstem connects to areas in the mid-brain, the cerebral core (not visible in Figure 1) which lies beneath the wrinkled outer layer of cortex. The mid-brain contains a lot of white matter (links between nerve cells) as well as grey matter (nerve cell bodies), often clustered into nuclei. Some of these nuclei, like the amygdala and thalamus, have been extensively studied, but most are still poorly understood.

Like the rest of the body, human brains have a left and a right half. The division is clearly visible at the level of the many mid-brain areas: there is a left and a right thalamus, hippocampus, amygdala, and so on. It is even more noticeable for cortex, whose left and right hemispheres are linked by a hefty bridge of fibres

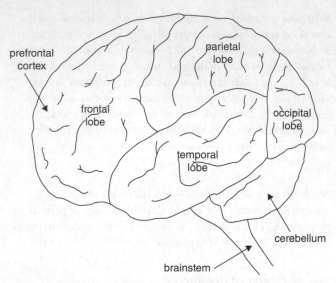

1. **The four lobes of the brain's cortex, seen from the outside.**

called the corpus callosum. Each cortical hemisphere is divided into four large lobes, marked out by natural grooves called sulci. Figure 1 shows the lobes for the left hemisphere. At the front of the brain, behind the forehead, is the frontal lobe, the foremost part of which is the prefrontal cortex. At the back is the occipital lobe, and at the sides the temporal lobe (lower) and parietal lobe (upper). Figure 1 also shows two major anatomical landmarks, one of which is the brainstem. The other is the cerebellum, tucked beneath the occipital lobe. The word cerebellum means 'little brain', and the cerebellum is involved with many key functions including emotion, attention, decision-making, and motor control.

Different lobes and areas seem to specialize in different kinds of cognition. Roughly—very roughly—the occipital lobe is concerned with vision, the parietal lobe with spatial awareness, movement detection, and the sense of having a body. The temporal lobe

14

tackles object recognition, hearing, memory, and emotional processing. The frontal lobe deals with decision-making, higher-level cognition (e.g. abstract thought and planning), moral and social judgements, and the regulation of behaviour. In dementia, neurodegeneration typically affects the temporal and frontal lobes earlier than the parietal or occipital lobes.

Figure 1 shows the brain's left hemisphere. What it does not show is that around the edges of both hemispheres, the cortical surface folds inward like a blanket tucked around the brain's core. These inner parts of cortex, hidden from view in a whole brain, can be seen in cross-section in Figure 2 (which represents how the brain would look if it were cut in half, slicing from top to bottom). Outer areas of cortex tend to process incoming data from outside the body, such as sights and sounds. Inner areas are more associated with internal, body-related stimuli, such as emotions and visceral signals. The latter come most notably from the vagus nerve, which carries messages from many body organs, like the heart and gut, via the brainstem.

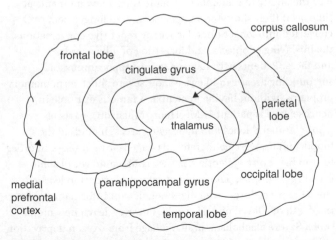

2. **The cortical lobes on the brain's inner surface.**

Figure 2 shows the inner parts of the four cortical lobes. It also shows the location of the corpus callosum, and of three other important brain areas: the thalamus, the cingulate gyrus, and the parahippocampal gyrus. (A gyrus is a ridge of brain tissue between two sulci.) The thalamus is where most of the signals from vision, hearing, and other senses come together for initial processing, before rushing off to the rest of the brain. The cingulate is crucial in the regulation of emotions, pain, attention, mood, motivation, and how well your innards work. And the parahippocampal gyrus, as the name suggests ('para' = 'around') is the cortex immediately surrounding the hippocampus, a structure key to memory and one of the most noticeable sites of damage in dementia.

The remembering brain

This whole area—the hippocampus and its cortical neighbourhood—is centrally involved in most cases of memory loss, cognitive decline, and dementia. Dementia patients often lose the ability to remember for more than a few moments at a time, as if their short-term memories are no longer being converted into longer ones. Hence the repetitive conversations, the mislaying of objects, and forgetting of bills, words, and faces. Patients with damage to the hippocampus and surrounding areas can likewise show severe short-term memory problems, without having dementia. A famous example in neuroscience is patient H.M. (Henry Molaison), parts of whose temporal lobes and underlying areas, including the hippocampus, were deliberately damaged—by surgery—in order to stop his severe epileptic seizures. H.M. could recall some pre-surgery events, but could not retain information learned since the procedure—even highly significant information, like the death of a loved one. He could, however, learn new motor skills. Severe alcoholism, brain damage from oxygen deprivation at birth, strokes, and brain infections can also cause hippocampal damage.

The hippocampus does not work like a computer memory or paper filing system. It seems to help with linking memories together for the long term, so that when one part of the memory is reactivated the rest can also be retrieved. This enables the person to, for instance, bite into a cake and have the taste conjure a vivid recollection of a distant time and place, coloured by the emotions they originally felt.

Yet that recalled memory does not stay pristine in the way a photograph would. Instead it is altered to fit with present circumstances. Imagine you have a memory of eating a certain cake just once in childhood, on a special occasion, say your tenth birthday. Then years later you eat biscuits with the same distinctive taste as part of having afternoon tea with friends. Later still, you may recall your tenth birthday treat as being in the afternoon, or remember someone drinking tea at it. These will feel like genuine recollections. Any memory is actually a composite of all the times when stimuli triggered the network of brain cells which is the physical basis of that memory—or parts of it. Thinking about a memory can subtly distort it. (This is why many eyewitness accounts in criminal cases turn out to be worthless, and why many people with brain disorders, including dementia, will state obvious falsehoods with sincerity, a symptom known as confabulation. Unless they have an ideology rather than a brain disease; then we call it propaganda.)

In dementia, as synapses fail, memories become less easy to retain and retrieve, and mis-linkages can become startlingly apparent. My relative's crossed wires—someone's American holiday becoming someone else's US residence—are an example.

The hippocampus is much more than a memory organ. It has roles in emotional processing, decision-making, and the resolving of internal conflicts and anxiety. It is a major regulator of the body's stress and other hormonal responses, with close links to the hypothalamus (governor of many vital functions, from appetite to aggression) and the amygdala (involved in social cognition and in processing emotions, especially fear and anxiety). Too much stress, psychological or physical, stops the hippocampus working properly. No wonder then that people under pressure often forget things, and that dementia symptoms worsen when patients are frightened, agitated, or physically unwell.

As I mentioned earlier, loss of the ability to recognize and steer through familiar environments is often an early sign of dementia, and the hippocampus is crucial in spatial navigation. Its structure allows recall of the environment, and routes through it, using the collective activity patterns of specialized 'place' and 'grid' cells. These construct map-like models of locations—but not in the neutral way we would expect of a human map, where real distances are reflected in the map's spacing. Instead, like a phone app highlighting your favourite walks or current route, the brain weights locations by their salience, giving them more prominence if they are of immediate interest or emotional significance. This allows the person to factor prior experience into their route planning. Losing this ability to apply knowledge, and to feel that a place is known, can lead to alarming disorientation and confusion.

These clinical symptoms appear long after the harm to, and death of, brain cells has begun. The human brain's immense adaptability allows it to compensate for many lost connections, and even for large numbers of dying cells, masking the severity of the damage. (This is how people can recover function after a stroke.) By the time a person is worried enough to have approached the medical profession and obtained a diagnosis of dementia, neurodegeneration will already be well under way.

Which cells are first affected varies. In ALS, it is the motor neurons which send command signals from the central nervous system to the body. In Parkinson's, neurons in a central area of the brain called the substantia nigra die off. In ataxia, the cerebellum (which regulates movements) and the brainstem (which connects the brain and spinal cord) are particularly affected. In Alzheimer's, parts of the brainstem may also be early targets, but the characteristic damage is found first in memory- and navigation-related structures like the hippocampus, which curls around the centre of the brain.

Most cases of dementia—about nineteen in every twenty—are sporadic: that is, their cause is not clearly genetic or caused by some known event or illness. They also tend to be late-onset; the risk rises sharply from pension age onwards (as discussed in Chapter 4 and shown in Figure 9). Even in sporadic cases, however, there is some effect of genes: having a parent with dementia does increase the chances of getting it yourself. Yet only rarely does dementia in the family ensure a high risk of younger members being affected. That occurs when there is a genetic mutation which, if inherited, will almost certainly inflict the illness. In such familial cases symptoms appear much earlier, while people are still working and, sometimes, parenting young children. Young-onset dementia is unusual, but what it lacks in frequency it more than makes up for in disruption. Those who have it must not only come to terms with the diagnosis, and rearrange their entire existence accordingly, but do so while pushing against the tide of expectation which thinks of dementia as something that happens to the old.

The costs of dementia

That research into neurodegeneration is still desperately needed, after several decades of intense study, may be disappointing, but it should not surprise us. The average human brain is thought to contain around 80 billion neurons, plus similar numbers of various other cells—known as glia—whose functions are only starting to be understood. Highly interconnected, these brain cells use thousands of interacting proteins and other chemicals. Most dementia cases cannot be traced to a single gene mutation, and even when they can, that mutation's effects are fearsomely complicated. There are numerous biochemical pathways involved, regulating many cell processes: growth, nutrition, and survival; protein formation, transport, and waste disposal; synaptic function and the neurotransmission of chemical signals between cells, and so on. If the key molecules implicated in, say, Alzheimer's had been found to interact with one or two such pathways we would probably have had good treatments for that disease by now. Unfortunately, those molecules seem to interact with all of them. This is why there is 'still' no cure for dementia: it is a fiendishly difficult problem.

Moreover, specimen brains for study are not easy to come by, making the research hard and expensive to do and slowing progress in understanding neurodegeneration. Donating one's body, or part of it, to medical research is not everyone's choice. Brain donation is done by a specialist system of brain banks (in the UK, contact the Human Tissue Authority for details), and it requires that the material is carefully preserved and treated as soon as possible after death. Thus plans for donation need to be thought through—and discussed with loved ones—well beforehand.

Funding is also an issue. Dementia research has been hugely underfunded compared with other major killers like heart disease and cancer. Even today, charitable giving in particular is far more likely to flow to cancer research—often to childhood cancers, which are rare (fewer than 2,000 cases diagnosed per year). A study of UK research funding, both governmental and charitable, for major diseases found that only three pounds in every hundred went to dementia science.

Yet dementia is an increasingly familiar cause of death. Globally, in 2017 it is thought to have killed more than twice as many people as breast, prostate, ovarian, and testicular cancer combined. Moreover, the number of people with dementia is growing fast as the world's population both increases and ages.

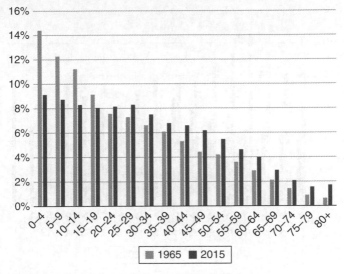

3. Changes in global population in the last half-century, as percentages by five-year age group.

Dementia risk rises sharply above age 60, and these days there are many more people at higher risk. In 1965, the United Nations (UN) estimated the global population of older people (60+) at almost 266 million, just under 8 per cent of the total. Fifty years later, in 2015, the number was 906 million, somewhat over 12 per cent. That's a massive demographic shift. (Regionally, the percentage varies from about 5 per cent in sub-Saharan Africa to about 24 per cent in Europe.)

Figures 3 and 4 show how the population has aged over the last half-century, comparing the percentage of the population in all five-year age groups up to age 80. Both figures plot data for 1965 (grey bars) and 2015 (black bars). Figure 3 represents data for the global population (from the UN). In 1965, the youngest ages (under 20) made up a much larger proportion than in 2015, which has more people in the older age groups. In both 1965 and 2015,

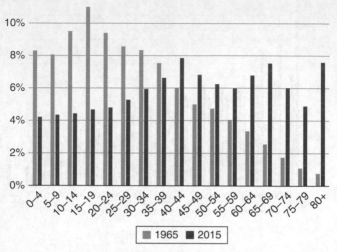

4. Changes in Japan's population in the last half-century, as percentages by five-year age group.

however, the downwards trend from youngest to oldest is similar from the mid-twenties upwards: older people make up a smaller segment of the population.

Figure 4 shows equivalent data for Japan, one of the nations where demographic ageing has been most noticeable. Again, there are relatively fewer young people in 2015 than fifty years earlier. However, the age distribution in Figure 4 is much flatter—even in 1965, and especially in 2015. (Note the different vertical scales in the two figures.) In the 1965 data (grey bars), you can still see a resemblance between the overall shape of the graph and the global data in Figure 3: larger numbers of young people (though not the very youngest); then the bars slope downward with increasing age. In the 2015 data the pattern is quite different, with far more older people. In 1965, just under a tenth of the Japanese population was 60 or over. In 2015, it was almost a third.

With health and social care systems already struggling, the interlinked problems of how to treat dementia, prevent it, and pay for its care costs are rising rapidly up the policy agenda. To have a chance of solving this gigantic problem, we will need to know more about what causes dementia. That is the topic of Chapter 2.

Chapter 2
What causes dementia?

This chapter looks at the mechanisms underlying dementia. The focus is on Alzheimer's, the best-known and most-researched type, but I will also mention other neurodegenerative disorders.

Alzheimer's findings

When Alois Alzheimer examined the withered brain of his patient Auguste D., he found distinctive signs of abnormality that are seen in many people with advanced dementia. The most obvious sign is that the brain is smaller, as if the disease has caused brain tissue to melt away. Even healthy brains lose cells as they get older—perhaps 10 per cent between ages 20 and 90. Brains affected by Alzheimer's disease, however, lose matter at rates which may be three times as fast as in healthy ageing. The loss of brain tissue can be stark, as Figure 5 shows.

Alzheimer also observed brain tissue marked with blotches of congealed material, varying in size up to about a third of a millimetre across. Often vaguely spherical in shape, like cerebral verrucas, these blotches, once called senile plaques, are now commonly known as amyloid plaques. Plaques form in the fluid-filled gaps between cells. They are fibrous clumps of proteins and other material, dominated by a protein called amyloid-beta.

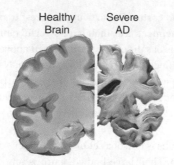

Healthy Brain   Severe AD

5. Brain changes in Alzheimer's (AD) compared with a healthy brain.

Since the gene that encodes it was identified in 1987, amyloid-beta has been central to research on Alzheimer's disease.

Alzheimer observed another abnormality, this time inside cells: thick strands of some tough material. As these 'fibrils' mature they form teardrop-shaped coils called neurofibrillary tangles which clog up, and eventually kill, brain cells. The fibrils are made of a protein called tau. Normally tau is a vital component of the cytoskeleton, the cell's internal scaffolding. Built from long rigid molecules, the cytoskeleton helps cells to keep their shape. It also provides a transport system for moving proteins made in the nucleus to distant regions like axons and synapses. When tau misfolds and gathers into tangles, it disrupts the cytoskeleton, harming and killing the cell's extremities first—including its synapses. Like amyloid plaques, tau tangles became a defining characteristic of Alzheimer's disease.

Beyond cortex

We now know that the cortex is not the only brain region affected in dementia, and not the first either. Evidence from human post-mortem studies suggests that neurodegeneration may begin deep down, spreading from the brainstem and mid-brain to the hippocampus and cortex. Of particular interest to people researching Alzheimer's is a small but powerful clump of cells called the nucleus basalis of Meynert, located above the optic nerve, which is affected very early in the disease. Named after the man who first described it—19th-century psychiatrist, anatomist, and poet Theodor Meynert—it is the brain's key source of a neurotransmitter called acetylcholine.

The nucleus basalis is one of a set of 'deep nuclei' with vital roles in brain function. Their large-bodied neurons send projections throughout the brain to influence its overall workings, from consciousness, alertness, and sleep to mood, motivation, and attention to incoming stimuli. Damage to the deep nuclei can cause symptoms ranging from apathy and lack of concentration to unconsciousness and coma. Unlike the cells in cortex, their main neurotransmitters are not glutamate and GABA. Instead they use other chemicals whose names have become familiar to many patients: serotonin (target of antidepressants like Prozac), dopamine (associated with reward, addiction, and Parkinson's), histamine (producer of misery for allergy sufferers), noradrenaline (*aka* norepinephrine, used to treat sepsis and heart attacks), as well as acetylcholine (ACh, which enables nerves to trigger muscle movements). All of these neurotransmitters, and the brain nuclei which use them, have been linked to dementia. The strongest connections to date are between Alzheimer's, ACh, and the nucleus basalis.

In Alzheimer's, brain levels of ACh drop early on. Large-scale studies have associated the use of common drugs which lower ACh levels—like amitriptyline (for depression) and some antihistamines (for allergies)—with a greater risk of cognitive problems and dementia, though the findings remain controversial. Post-mortem examinations of brains from people of different ages have found that the nucleus basalis shows signs of damage in younger brains than does the cortex. Stimulating the nucleus basalis electrically can boost short-term memory in monkeys. And some research suggests that acetylcholinesterase, the protein which breaks down ACh after use, can generate a toxic protein fragment capable of damaging brain cells. Reducing levels of this toxin, and boosting levels of ACh, can both be done by blocking acetylcholinesterase—and this has so far been the most successful treatment strategy in dementia. Of the four standard drugs used to slow the progression of the illness, donepezil (also known as Aricept), galantamine (Reminyl), and rivastigmine (Exelon) are all acetylcholinesterase inhibitors.

These drugs, which have been around for decades, are undoubtedly useful, but they are nowhere near a cure. Many scientists soon began to look elsewhere for hypotheses that might lead to better treatments. With technological advances to boost new research, they returned to the most noticeable signs identified by Alois Alzheimer—plaques—and focused their attention on what was in those blotchy, verrucous clusters. Asking that question led to the most influential theory to date of what causes dementia: the amyloid cascade hypothesis.

Sticky proteins

Amyloid proteins, of which there are many, are fascinating entities. In ways we still don't fully understand, they can take a wide range of shapes and functions, and perform many useful tasks in the brain and body. Small changes in protein production, however, can boost levels of 'misfolded' proteins, and this is what happens with amyloid-beta in Alzheimer's (see Figure 6).

Amyloid proteins, especially when misfolded, like to stick together. Literally. Individual proteins, known as monomers, gather into oligomers, and these in turn can link up to form—well, polymers, you might think, but that name was already taken. Instead, longer strands of amyloid-beta are called proto-fibrils,

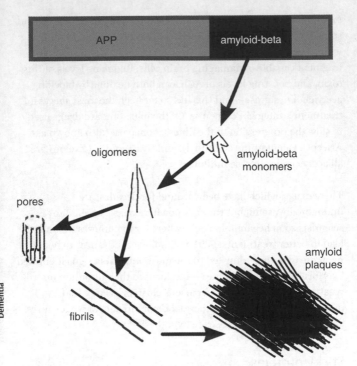

6. APP processing gives rise to various formats of amyloid-beta.

and they in turn accumulate into fibrils. These clump together to form sheets of material which amalgamate into plaques. Oligomers can also form tube-like structures called pores. These can punch holes in cell membranes, weakening or even destroying the cell.

As the amyloid collective grows, it solidifies. Monomers and oligomers are soluble; fibrils and plaques are not. So smaller units of amyloid proteins can behave very differently from larger ones. The size depends on how much protein there is in the area. Like salt crystals growing in salted water, amyloids cluster into solids at higher concentrations.

To make matters even more complicated, the amyloid-beta protein comes in different lengths, and behaves differently depending on how many amino acids it has. For example, the type of amyloid-beta thought to dominate in Alzheimer's (which has forty-two amino acids) may have more toxic oligomers, and is more prone to form plaques, than the type associated with vascular dementia (which has forty amino acids).

Alzheimer used cell staining to highlight plaques in dead brain tissue. Current techniques can detect them in living brains. Detecting the smaller, soluble oligomers, however, is proving trickier. This matters because many researchers think that it is oligomers, not plaques, which are the most important players in Alzheimer's disease.

The amyloid cascade

Why does Alzheimer's disease have such a profound impact on brain function and structure? For years now, the leading scientific answer to this question has been the amyloid cascade hypothesis. First fully set out in 1992 by John Hardy and Gerald Higgins, in the high-profile journal *Science*, this hypothesis sees amyloid-beta as the central problem in Alzheimer's. The key claim is that too much amyloid protein builds up in the brain, and that this then causes whatever else goes wrong.

Today, the field of Alzheimer's research divides into those who support the amyloid cascade hypothesis, with modifications, and those who think too much time and money has already been spent on it—with the latter group increasing in recent years. In Chapter 3, I will look at their criticisms. However, there is also considerable evidence for the hypothesis, and many scientists still favour some version of it. This is at least in part because the core idea is so attractively simple and optimistic. If a single protein were the root cause, successful drug treatments would only need to interfere with that protein.

How has this powerful idea been tested? The science of dementia has always depended on four key areas: animal research, human tissue samples, living patients and their families, and technological advances in neuroscience and beyond.

Animal studies

Animal research has taught scientists a huge amount about how brains age, and the changes that occur during neurodegeneration. Many experiments are done on simpler species like yeast, worms, and fruit flies, which are quickly and easily bred. Their cells have a lot of biochemical pathways in common with ours, and the networks of interactions can be analysed in great detail. Mice and rats have brains and behaviours more similar to humans, but experiments take longer, and the systems being studied are more complicated.

Most research on dementia does not involve animals. Of that which does, only a tiny minority involves more controversial species such as primates.

Human samples

Human tissue samples traditionally came from people who had generously donated their bodies to research. Post-mortem samples have always been central to research, and remain so in the current age of advanced genetic and molecular biological techniques. However, brain samples are in short supply, and sometimes preservation methods may damage tissue. Also, the donor may have been ill, or donations may not be representative of the population. (Every method has its limitations; that's why scientists use so many methods.)

One recent advance, made possible by growing knowledge of how cells develop, involves stem cells and organoids. Stem cells, which grow in bone marrow, are the source of replacements for the body's short-lived cells (blood cells, for instance, only last about three months). Stem cells have the potential to become any one of multiple cell types, depending on what chemical signals they receive.

Most cells, by contrast, are 'fate-restricted'. They have developed the fixed characteristics of a skin cell, neuron, or whatever, and are no longer capable of changing into anything else—in the body. However, scientists can now reprogramme fate-restricted cells, converting them first to stem cells, then to another cell type. Thus cells can be taken from a person's skin or blood and transformed into brain cells. This offers a non-invasive way of obtaining brain-like samples, personalized to the individual's particular genetic code. And provided the person's original sample is stored safely, the transformation can be done at any time. It can even take place after their death, once it is known for sure exactly which kind of illness they had. This is no use to the individual, of course; but it does help researchers to understand their illness more precisely, and thus to develop better treatments.

Organoids are clusters of cells grown on a 3D scaffold. They were developed to build organs for transplantation, in order to overcome the problem of the recipient's immune system rejecting the donation. However, the technique is now being used to grow segments of brain tissue—mini-brains. These can include neurons, glial cells, and blood vessels, and are used to study interactions between these different cell types. They bring researchers closer to actual brain function. (Indeed, some are already worrying about how to tell if a mini-brain is conscious.)

Living people

Patients and their families are critically important for dementia research, since dementia cannot be modelled adequately in either animals or mini-brains. Some of the strongest evidence for the amyloid cascade hypothesis comes from studying families with early-onset dementia. Studying patients with less clearly genetic forms of the illness has also been extremely informative, as have healthy individuals, both young and old. Healthy volunteers are essential controls for experimental trials. They can also be studied over long periods to assess how dementia first develops. Many thousands of people have taken part in such research.

Large-scale studies are invaluable for identifying risk factors for dementia and early warning signs. Some of these studies are cross-sectional: this involves sampling a group at one moment in time, collecting lots of data on them, and looking at which factors seem to go together (e.g. diet and current cognitive function). Other studies are prospective: the experiment's aims are set out in advance, participants gathered and assessed, and then researchers wait to see how they change over time (e.g. how many of them get dementia). Prospective studies are generally more useful and reliable, but they are also more expensive and take longer to produce results.

Finally, patients provide crucial assistance to researchers and clinicians by volunteering to test drugs and other treatments.

Technological advances

Smart methods are essential to scientific progress, and the science of dementia has benefited greatly from developments elsewhere, including: improved computing and the statistics to analyse big data; work on the human genome and quicker, cheaper genotyping; advances in electrode technology to make recording brain electrical signals more accurate; and better ways of storing and preparing samples such as brain slices.

The revolution in genetics and molecular biology has also enabled researchers to develop immensely useful animal models in which one or more genes have been precisely modified. Such changes can boost the amount of a single protein, or prevent its production;

genetically modified and healthy animals can then be compared. Mice used in dementia research are often genetically modified to alter, for example, how their brains process amyloid, or to carry mutations found in families with early-onset illness. New technologies are also allowing scientists to learn much more about how, where, and when particular genes are expressed in brain cells.

Among the best-known neuroscience technologies are the various types of neuroimaging methods—brain scans. Clinically, people are most likely to encounter these in the form of CT or MRI scans. CT (computer tomography) scans are fancy X-rays: they combine multiple images taken at different locations around the head to make a 3D picture of the brain. MRI (magnetic resonance imaging) scans can be used to infer the type of matter in an area (structural MRI); they can 'see' changes such as tissue loss, tumours, problems with white matter, or damage to blood vessels. MRI can also be used to detect changes in blood flow (functional MRI, fMRI), which reflects the brain's electromagnetic activity. This shows which areas are working harder, or less hard, than they should be, for example during an epileptic seizure or memory test.

MRI scanning has transformed neuroscience, but it has its limitations. It requires powerful magnets and can induce claustrophobia. Moreover, although changes in blood flow track the electromagnetic shifts of a living brain, they do so somewhat sluggishly. To get round this, scientists record the electromagnetic signals directly. MEG, magnetoencephalography, measures the brain's magnetic fields. EEG, electroencephalography, measures its electrical signals. You may encounter these methods if you volunteer for a research study.

The other major neuroimaging technique is PET, positron emission tomography. It fell out of fashion as MRI developed, but it is now proving extremely useful in studying neurodegenerative disorders. This is because, unlike MRI, PET can 'see' where molecules of interest—such as tau or amyloid-beta—are located in the brain. It can be used to detect a wide range of molecules; and since different cells have different chemicals on their surfaces, it can also pick out particular types of cell. PET involves making a mildly radioactive form of the molecule of interest, or of a chemical which will bind to it. This radioactive 'tracer' is then administered to a volunteer, so that it gets into their brain. There, the PET scanner can detect and localize the particles emitted as the radioactivity decays.

Biomarkers

MRI and PET are now being used to study amyloid-beta and other amyloid proteins. This has allowed researchers and clinicians to observe how heavily laden a brain is with amyloid deposits. Such deposits are a possible 'biomarker' for dementia.

Disease biomarkers are physiological features, such as genes or levels of blood proteins, which reliably discriminate individuals with the disease from healthy people. To be effective, biomarkers should do this across many different human groups, using widely available techniques and with as little trauma as possible. Ideally, biomarkers should occur only in, or before, the illness in question, and not in healthy people, nor in those with other medical conditions. In other words, what researchers and doctors want is a simple test with high sensitivity—it is good at detecting when the disease is present—and high specificity—it efficiently rules out people who do not have that disease.

As technologies develop, so do biomarkers. In cancer, for example, scientists can now detect genetic markers of the disease—fragments of DNA and RNA which have detached from the tumour and floated off into the bloodstream. This is especially important for types such as pancreatic and ovarian cancer, whose early stages have few symptoms or whose symptoms are easily mistaken for less urgent problems. Such tests for genetic biomarkers are already being used, though they are not yet as accurate as doctors would like. Once the tests can detect the fragments without confusing them with other, similar, normal proteins, this will allow cancer patients to be identified and treated faster. That should lessen the negative impact of treatment as well as sparing healthy people the shock of being misdiagnosed.

Biomarkers are desirable because they can be repeatedly and reliably measured, and do not rely on a person's report or subjective memory. Indeed—as with the genetic fragments in cancer—the patient may not be aware of them: they are clinical signs of illness, not noticed symptoms. Thus they can be used to predict the presence (or likely occurrence) of a disease even when the patient has no clinical symptoms and feels well, sometimes years before the disease takes hold.

Possible biomarkers for dementia visible with brain scanning include not only amyloid deposits, but measures of tau and other brain proteins implicated in neurodegeneration. Scans can also measure a brain's glucose consumption (energy use), as well as its structure, white matter, volume, and activity. From a brain's activity, scientists can infer its connectivity—how well various regions talk to each other. Changes in connectivity are an early result of damage to synapses and white matter, and may precede more obvious loss of grey matter.

Other biomarkers include measures of amyloid-beta or related proteins in saliva, blood, or cerebrospinal fluid (CSF). Often a ratio is taken, for example of short vs longer forms of amyloid-beta. Researchers are also investigating the use of non-invasive techniques, such as retinal imaging—already used in conditions like diabetes—to detect amyloid deposits around blood vessels in the eye.

All of these techniques have advantages and disadvantages. Mouth swabs, eye scans, or blood tests are easier, quicker, and cheaper than neuroimaging. CT scans are quicker than fMRI or PET scans, but less informative. Lumbar punctures and tissue biopsies are painfully invasive; but amyloid-beta levels in the CSF (which bathes the brain) differ from levels in other body fluids, so sampling blood or saliva may not shed enough light on brain amyloid. Scans detect plaques, but not (yet) the more dangerous oligomers, nor other proteins of interest. There are questions about how specific the chemicals used in PET scans really are. And so on.

These problems are not insuperable. Recent studies suggest that amyloid-beta blood measures may be clinically useful, while eye scans are showing promise as an early diagnostic tool. Biomarkers are also proving useful in clinical trials involving people with dementia, not least because they can help researchers to check their volunteers have sufficiently similar neurodegenerative conditions to provide a homogeneous group for study. This is especially important given the difficulties of diagnosing Alzheimer's and other dementias.

Incidentally, biomarkers do not need to be physiological. For example, cognitive tests which produce objective measures of performance could be used if their scores changed reliably with disease severity. An example would be tests of spatial navigation, such as finding one's way through a virtual landscape or maze. Indeed, a citizen science project has used smartphone technology to study this ability by inviting participants to play a video game called *Sea Hero Quest*.

These methods and others have transformed the science of dementia. As we shall see, they have supported, changed, and challenged the amyloid cascade hypothesis. To understand how, we first need to learn a little about that hypothesis, and about how amyloid-beta is made and processed in the brain.

Making amyloid-beta

Amyloid-beta protein does not have its own gene. Instead, the DNA codes for a much larger molecule called amyloid precursor protein (APP); this *APP* gene is the one identified in 1987. (By convention, gene names are written in italics.) Three years earlier, US researchers George Glenner and Caine Wong reported that they had purified the amyloid-beta protein.

APP was so-called because at the time no one knew what it did, apart from making (being a precursor of) amyloid-beta. Subsequent research has shown, however, that APP is useful in its own right. Good for brain cells, it facilitates learning and helps neurons, synapses, and dendrites to flourish. It may even protect neurons against lack of oxygen (hypoxia), one of the most damaging effects of stroke.

Humans have three forms of APP, ranging in length from 695 to 770 amino acids. Amyloid-beta is much smaller—its two major forms contain forty and forty-two amino acids—and must be cut out from APP by specialized proteins: enzymes. How the cutting is done determines how much amyloid-beta is made, what shape it ends up being, and thus how readily it aggregates into oligomers, fibrils, pores, and plaques.

Genes predispose us to certain illnesses, including dementia. Whether we get sick, however, also depends on what happens to proteins after their production.

APP, like all proteins, is made when DNA is 'read off' to form RNA (transcription), and that RNA is matched with amino acids to assemble a protein string (translation). But that is just the start. To produce the three-dimensional structures which do so many jobs in cells, the amino-acid strings are hacked about, tagged with various chemicals, and folded up in complicated ways. How they are folded affects what they then do. This cellular origami—known as 'post-translation processing'—happens in a cell's central area, in and around the nucleus where DNA is stored.

From the nucleus, the newly folded APP is carried to the cell's boundary, its membrane. Pushed through the membrane like a kebab stick through a chunk of food, it protrudes outside—into the extracellular fluid—and inside—into the cell. Both ends attract enzymes called secretases which act like scissors, chopping off large segments of APP (see Figure 7).

Without this chemical sculpting, amyloid-beta would remain embedded within APP, unable to escape into the extracellular

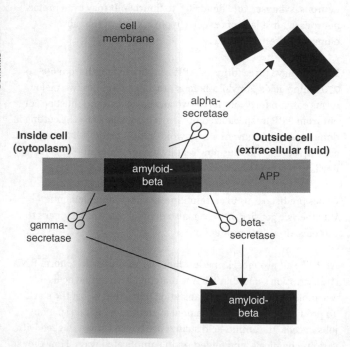

7. **How amyloid-beta is extracted from APP.**

fluid and fraternize with its fellow proteins. But its release is not inevitable.

Secretases outside the cell act first. There are two of these, alpha- and beta-secretase, and they cut through APP in different places; but only one of them can cut each APP molecule. This matters because if alpha-secretase strikes first it cuts APP at a point in the middle of the embedded amyloid-beta, destroying it before it can be released. Beta-secretase, however, bites through APP at one end of the amyloid-beta molecule. Then a third enzyme, gamma-secretase, acts inside the cell to sever APP at the other, inner end, allowing amyloid-beta to escape. So whether alpha- or beta-secretase acts first determines whether amyloid-beta is produced; and this depends on how much of each secretase is available.

Some APP molecules are retrieved from the membrane before they are dismembered, and sent for recycling. This is another way of regulating amyloid-beta production, since alpha-secretase is mostly found at the membrane, whereas beta-secretase is also common in cells' internal recycling areas. Thus APP sent for recycling is more prone to be converted into amyloid-beta. This is more likely to happen when the cell is stressed—for example, by hypoxia or the wear and tear of ageing.

In other words, amyloid production is not something that just happens, but a tightly regulated sequence of events. For evolution to have developed such complex control of a biochemical process—akin to what is seen in the immune system—suggests two things about amyloid-beta production. First, it is biologically important. Secondly, it may be dangerous.

Amyloid-beta is made by brain cells, but they are not its only source. One of the most interesting recent developments in neuroscience is the growing realization that other body organs, like the gut, the liver, and the immune system, have a powerful impact on how well the brain works. We will look at the immune system in due course. As for the gut, its tissues make amyloid-beta, which can get into the brain—or out of it, whereupon it circulates in the blood. Like other proteins, when it reaches the liver it is broken down for recycling, if the liver is healthy.

Dysfunction in other organs, like the lungs and kidneys, is also increasingly linked to neurodegeneration, and this is changing how scientists perceive dementia. It used to be seen as a mental illness, caused by a brain disorder. These days it is looking more and more like a whole-body problem. Science is catching up with what people living with dementia have long known.

Getting rid of amyloid-beta

If, as the amyloid cascade hypothesis proposes, too much amyloid-beta is being produced in Alzheimer's, then reducing production would be one approach to treatment. Another would involve boosting the brain's own sophisticated mechanisms for removing unwanted proteins. These include pushing the material out into the blood for the liver to crunch, washing it out through specialized sewage systems, breaking it down using enzymes, or encouraging brain cells to eat it.

Brain cells are expert at protein management. Unfortunately, age is the biggest risk factor for dementia, and the wear and tear that comes with age damages DNA and makes many cellular processes less effective. Among them is waste disposal. DNA damage can cause errors in the manufacture of proteins—including the enzymes which chop up amyloid-beta. Toxins and pollutants in the blood can get into cells and damage their proteins—including the intricate network of enzymes which controls protein trafficking and waste management. And gene mutations which reduce this network's effectiveness have been linked to a greater risk of dementia. Some such mutations are known to cause other neurodegenerative disorders, like ataxia.

Neurons can ingest and destroy amyloid-beta, as long as there is not too much of it to swallow. So can other brain cells, notably astrocytes and microglia. These are types of glial cells, which make up about half of the brain's cells. Glia were traditionally viewed as cerebral servants, dancing attendance on the more glamorous neurons. We now know better: both astrocytes and microglia have crucial roles in brain function. Astrocytes have their own electrochemical communication networks, as well as interacting with neurons; they also help regulate brain water levels, acidity, and much else besides. (One of the deadliest brain diseases, glioblastoma multiforme, occurs when astrocytes turn cancerous. It is rare—1–2 cases per 100,000 people—but near-impossible to treat.) Microglia are the brain's resident immune cells, defending against infection and other hazards.

As well as brain cells eating amyloid-beta, there are also enzymes in the extracellular fluid which can cut it up; and two of these are important for other reasons. One, insulin-degrading enzyme, breaks down insulin, the key regulator of blood sugar. The second, angiotensin-converting enzyme, activates the hormone angiotensin, which raises blood pressure. Angiotensin is also thought to affect brains in ways which could encourage neurodegeneration, so like insulin (and amyloid-beta) it requires tight control, which may slip in ageing brains. If more amyloid-beta is present, these enzymes are more likely to be occupied with degrading it, rather than controlling insulin and angiotensin levels.

Likewise, potential treatments for Alzheimer's need to be careful not to interfere with these enzymes. Disruption to either blood glucose or blood pressure management can cause serious illness, or, in extreme cases, death.

This is one reason why developing treatments based on the amyloid cascade hypothesis has proved much more difficult than expected. Because amyloid-beta processing is intertwined with that of insulin, angiotensin, and many other important molecules, some would-be drugs have either not worked as expected, or have had very serious side-effects.

The genetics of dementia

Unsurprisingly, the genes for APP and for the alpha-, beta-, and gamma-secretases have been of enormous interest to researchers working on Alzheimer's. (The altruistic volunteering of families affected by early-onset inherited dementia has been immensely helpful to researchers, allowing them to identify genetic mutations and learn much about their effects.) Gamma-secretase, for example, is built from four proteins. Two of these, presenilin (PSEN) 1 and PSEN2, were named because of their clear link to early-onset ('presenile') dementia, and are key to how the secretase works.

Mutations in these genes can have a terrible impact. One 2017 study (by Lou and colleagues, listed in the References section) reports the case of a young man with a mutated *PSEN1* gene. His first symptoms—affecting his walking—appeared at age 23. By age 24 he was showing not only motor symptoms but visual impairment and cognitive difficulties with speech, memory, and knowing where and when he was. He also experienced apathy, personality change, problems with eating, and incontinence.

For later-onset dementia cases where there is no such obvious mutation, individual genetic variation is still important. Some people's biochemical mechanisms work better than others even at younger ages. For example, how effectively amyloid-beta is shuttled in and out of the brain, and broken down within it, depends on a protein called apolipoprotein E (APOE). Apolipoproteins carry fats such as cholesterol around the bloodstream, and APOE is the predominant fat-transporter in the brain. It also binds to amyloid-beta and stimulates its production. It is by far the biggest genetic risk factor for late-onset dementia.

In humans the *APOE* gene has three possible forms, or alleles: *APOE2*, *APOE3*, or *APOE4*. Since each of us inherits one allele from each parent, and since these can be the same or different, we have either one or two variants of the APOE protein. The difference between the variants affects only two of APOE's 299 amino acids, but the impact on dementia risk is enormous. It is thought that around one in every seven people (around 14 per cent) carries a copy of the *APOE4* allele. Among patients with Alzheimer's, the proportion with *APOE4* is much higher, around 60–80 per cent. Relative to inheriting the most common allele, *APOE3*, from both parents, having two copies of *APOE4* may boost dementia risk by between ten and thirty times. (The estimates vary because they are done in different populations. Higher risks have been found in Caucasian, Chinese, and Japanese people, lower risks in black Africans.)

APOE4 has also been implicated in vascular dementia and in other illnesses, including coronary heart disease, haemorrhagic stroke (brain bleeds), and late-life depression. It may worsen outcomes after brain injury, give a poorer prognosis to multiple sclerosis, and even increase susceptibility to CJD. *APOE2*, the rarest allele, can also lead to medical problems—such as atherosclerosis, high levels of blood fats, and complications of type two diabetes—but having *APOE2* greatly reduces the chance of getting dementia. However, it has been linked to other forms of neurodegeneration involving tau protein abnormalities. Having two copies of *APOE3* thus appears to be the safest option.

Interestingly, a rare mutated form of *APOE3* has recently been reported in a woman who began having cognitive problems in her seventies. Why is that noteworthy? Because she belongs to an extended (and much-studied) family with a *PSEN1* mutation that causes young-onset dementia. She has the mutation, which normally affects people in their forties, yet has lived without ill-effects for three decades longer. More research is needed, but it looks as if the change to her two *APOE3* alleles could be the source of this remarkable delay.

The APOE protein carries not only cholesterol but other blood fats like triglycerides and phospholipids to cells that need them. Triglycerides can be used as fuel; cholesterol and phospholipids are essential for cell membranes. People with APOE4 have less efficient cholesterol transport. APOE4 is more likely than the other variants to form LDL particles (low-density lipoprotein) than HDL (high-density lipoprotein); and LDL is heavy on triglycerides, while HDL is rich in cholesterol. LDL, sometimes called 'bad cholesterol', is prone to clog up blood vessels and cause dangerous inflammation of vessel walls—potentially leading to atherosclerosis. HDL, so-called 'good cholesterol', helps to damp down inflammation.

Compared with other variants, APOE4 is thought to boost amyloid-beta transport into the brain, while reducing its removal to the blood. It also reduces the ability of brain cells like microglia to ingest and destroy amyloid protein.

Small but deadly

Searching for clues in Auguste Deter's brain, Alois Alzheimer saw amyloid plaques. However, scientists now think that the smaller, soluble oligomers are the most toxic form of amyloid-beta. Studies suggest that they can damage synapses: reducing the plasticity that allows for learning, altering levels of important proteins, and even, when they form pores, puncturing the cells' membranes. Since cells depend on firm border control, in order to maintain the chemical gradients between inside and outside, this can be life-threatening.

Punctures disrupt how synapses work—and many other cell processes as well—by allowing the inflow of charged molecules, especially calcium. Calcium is a dangerous molecule in excess, and is normally kept on a very tight rein. Too much of it first overstimulates, then damages, and finally destroys the cell. As neurodegeneration takes hold, there is often a temporary surge in neural activity, similar to the frenetic over-signalling seen in epilepsy: excess calcium is thought to be responsible in both cases. Indeed, one hypothesis about why neurodegeneration takes hold proposes calcium as the key cause of cell damage. Of the four drugs commonly used to treat Alzheimer's, three, as mentioned earlier, affect acetylcholine. But the fourth, memantine, interferes with glutamate transmission, which involves calcium.

Amyloid-beta oligomers have also been implicated in many other types of cell damage, from interfering with the production of key proteins to harmful effects on membranes and mitochondria. These effects are not yet fully understood, despite decades of effort. Amyloid-beta is a hard molecule to work with in the lab. It's a slippery shape-shifter which comes in different lengths, shapes, and toxicities, its character changing depending on how it is analysed. Its interactions with other brain chemicals are also extremely complicated, and still being unravelled.

This complexity is why earlier hopes of a short and simple search for Alzheimer's treatments have evaporated. Yet for many researchers, blocking amyloid's harm before it becomes irreversible remains the best hope for combating the illness.

Backing amyloid

Much evidence supports the amyloid hypothesis. Experiments on cell samples and animals show that amyloid-beta can damage cells and synapses. Administering the protein to animals via the blood, or directly into the brain, can lead to the kinds of neurodegenerative damage seen in human brains with Alzheimer's. In animal models of Alzheimer's disease, lowering amyloid levels can reduce both the physical damage and behavioural signs of cognitive impairment.

In humans, as we have seen, the genetics of early-onset dementia are closely linked to amyloid-beta processing. To date, all known mutations for inherited Alzheimer's involve either the protein from which amyloid-beta is made, APP, or the gamma-secretase enzyme which releases it. A mutation which reduces levels of amyloid-beta production has been found to protect against Alzheimer's. Additional evidence comes from Down's syndrome, in which amyloid deposits start appearing early—sometimes in the teens—and dementia usually follows. Down's is caused by an extra copy of chromosome 21, which includes the *APP* gene. In late-onset dementia, the strongest genetic influence identified so far, *APOE*, also influences amyloid's actions in the brain.

Levels of APP and amyloid-beta in blood and CSF can distinguish between healthy people, those with mild cognitive impairment, and those with dementia. Brain scans can pick up amyloid deposits—between cells and around blood vessels—which typically increase with age; these are more extensive in people with worse cognitive function, vascular dementia, and Alzheimer's. And many of the risk factors for dementia appear to interact with amyloid processing.

Establishing causality is more difficult. Animal models of dementia are not the same as the human illness; and whatever your view of animal research, it is clearly unethical to give amyloid-beta to people and see whether they go on to get dementia.

Adding amyloids

The core of the amyloid cascade hypothesis is the idea that too much amyloid protein leads to the formation of aggregates harmful to the brain. Support for the proposed mechanism comes from the growing recognition that amyloid-beta is not the only amyloid. Other abnormally aggregating proteins are also linked to diseases which, like Alzheimer's, get gradually worse and eventually kill.

In the body, for example, amyloid aggregates can cause a disease called systemic amyloidosis, in which clumps of protein clog up organs until they can no longer function. One well-known victim of this disease, for anyone interested in UK and Irish politics, was Martin McGuinness, the controversial Sinn Fein politician and former IRA commander who helped to steer his country away from the Troubles. Amyloidosis also killed George Glenner, whose 1984 report of the purification of amyloid-beta was foundational for modern dementia research.

In the brain, we now know there are numerous kinds of amyloid protein, each with its own particular pattern of damage. Besides amyloid-beta, we have already come across the one Alzheimer himself observed: the misfolded tau that forms neurofibrillary tangles. Tau tangles are particularly prominent in frontotemporal dementia, as well as in Alzheimer's and Pick's disease. They are also found after severe brain injury, in the cognitive dysfunction and dementia resulting from contact sports, and in the rarer neurodegenerative disorders progressive supranuclear palsy and corticobasal degeneration. As Alzheimer's patient showed him, more than one protein can misfold and aggregate in a single brain.

In Parkinson's and in DLB a key culprit is a protein called alpha-synuclein, thought to help regulate neurotransmitter release (Lewy bodies are deposits of alpha-synuclein that accumulate inside neurons). In some forms of motor neuron disease, the chief suspect is called TDP-43 and helps to regulate DNA function (TDP-43 is also implicated in dementia). In other forms of ALS, it is called superoxide dismutase and helps protect cells against wear and tear. In Huntington's disease, the mutated protein was named for the disease—huntingtin. In some forms of dementia it is a multitasking protein, progranulin; in some forms of ataxia, a waste disposal regulator, josephin. And so on.

47

The most notorious example is surely prion protein, which causes CJD. Like Alzheimer's, this disease can be caused by genetic mutations—in the gene for prion protein—or it can be sporadic. The sporadic type, known as 'variant Creutzfeldt-Jakob', vCJD, came to prominence in Britain in the 1980s, due to people eating meat from cows infected with the prion disease BSE (bovine spongiform encephalopathy, 'mad cow disease'). Until the 1980s, British cattle were often fed meat and bone meal made from other cows. Since some were infected with prions, this allowed BSE to spread through the nation's herds, creating an enormously expensive—and alarming—health scare. BSE was officially recognized as a disease in 1986, and peaked in the early 1990s. By the time the crisis was contained millions of cattle had been slaughtered and billions of pounds lost from the UK economy. Over 150 people were known to have contracted vCJD. Cases, though thankfully rare, are still occurring, as the interval between infection and the disease making itself known can be decades-long.

Prion diseases like vCJD show how dangerous amyloid proteins can be—and raise the alarming prospect that other amyloid disorders could be infectious. Under certain conditions, it seems that amyloid proteins can indeed spread through cells, thanks to a remarkable property called 'seeding' or 'templating'. Added to a cell, the amyloid molecules can trigger the production of new copies of the misfolded protein, which then travel, virus-like, to nearby cells. Prion protein, tau, TDP-43, alpha-synuclein, and amyloid-beta have all been shown to do this in cells and in animal models.

As was found with prion disease, amyloids are physically tough and hard to destroy with normal sterilization methods. In vCJD, prions have been found to infect people not only via food but through medical routes, such as surgery with inadequately cleaned instruments, blood transfusion, corneal transplants, or the practice of giving human growth hormone to children deemed deficient in it. Transfer via pregnancy has also been known. Fortunately, vCJD is rare. We do not yet know whether amyloid-beta, tau, and other amyloids can spread in the same ways as prion protein. Patients infected with CJD via medical treatments, such as growth hormone recipients, have shown unexpectedly high levels of amyloid-beta pathology, suggesting that they might have developed Alzheimer's had they lived long enough. However, animal experiments with more everyday routes of transmission, such as close contact, have so far found no evidence to support the idea that amyloid-beta, or Alzheimer's, could be passed from one person to another.

Why would human bodies have evolved such dangerous proteins? That is not yet fully understood, but amyloids are not always problematic. The ability to knit together into larger structures has its uses: in healing wounds, for instance, or when quarantining dangerous toxins. Some researchers think that amyloid plaques can act as reservoirs, soaking up and storing potentially harmful chemicals like iron and copper—and perhaps the more toxic amyloid-beta oligomers—which would otherwise damage the brain. And at least one kind of amyloid, involving the protein TDP-43, is now thought to be essential for skeletal muscles, according to a 2018 study.

And yet, no cure

The amyloid cascade hypothesis has come to dominate research into dementia. Many years of time, and vast amounts of money, have been spent pursuing it, leading to well over 100 clinical trials of drugs which interfere with amyloid-beta processing. Some of these, such as the gamma-secretase inhibitor semagacestat and certain drugs inhibiting beta-secretase (also known as BACE inhibitors), have tried to stop the brain making amyloid. Other trials have attempted to lower its levels. For example, newer immunotherapy approaches have used vaccination methods: stimulating antibodies which will attach to amyloid-beta and remove it, as if it were a virus. Alongside the hunt for a successful treatment, researchers have learned an immense amount about how brain cells manage—or fail to manage—proteins.

Unfortunately, and despite apparent effectiveness in animals, none of these trials has yet produced a cure, or even a treatment. Some, like semagacestat, actually made symptoms worse by interfering with other important proteins in the brain. The lack of clinical advances is causing some scientists to look for alternatives to the amyloid hypothesis. Others continue to support some variant of it. In Chapter 3, we'll take a look at these reactions, and venture beyond amyloid.

Chapter 3
Beyond amyloid

This chapter looks at challenges to the amyloid cascade hypothesis of Alzheimer's disease. It has come to dominate dementia research; but that success has not been matched in the clinic. Critics point out that, as people seek to explain why drug trials have failed, the amyloid hypothesis has become more complicated. Some fear it might head the way of Ptolemy's Earth-centred theory of planetary motion: tweaked and patched beyond plausibility.

There are other criticisms. One is that the hypothesis has sucked too much attention away from other areas, leading researchers to focus less on the study of dementia—a condition suffered by people—than the study of amyloid—a material produced by brain cells. As scientists delve ever deeper into biochemical details, with ever more advanced methods, do they risk forgetting about the human beings they are being funded to help?

Another worry is that undue focus on amyloid-beta may be drowning out other interesting approaches with more promise for treatment. Funding is a very limited resource, and even science has its fashions. If the senior academics in a research field have all built their careers around one hypothesis they may, understandably, be reluctant to pay attention to competing ideas.

Yet times are changing. The US National Institutes of Health (NIH) is now spending more than half of its Alzheimer's budget (of around $2 billion) on topics other than tau and amyloid-beta. And when NIH changes direction, other funders take note.

Of mice and humans

Concerns have also been raised about the genetic evidence cited in favour of the amyloid hypothesis. Much of the work depends on research done in mice; but even very elderly mice do not naturally seem to get mouse Alzheimer's. Like many other species, they have a difference in their *APP* gene which, though only slight, is enough to stop their brains from making amyloid in the same way human brains do. To be useful models, the mice must be genetically engineered to incorporate DNA for human-format APP.

Transgenic mouse models which over-produce amyloid-beta have taught scientists a vast amount—about amyloid-beta—but they are problematic. Of course, animal experiments are inevitably controversial on ethical grounds. But it is also not clear how good the transgenic models are—how closely they resemble human Alzheimer's. Mice don't have language, so can't complain about forgetting things and feeling disoriented. Instead they are assessed on how well they learn and remember, or find their way round mazes. Yet despite forgetting things and getting lost, transgenic mice struggle to reproduce the behavioural and anatomical patterns of human dementia. They also produce amyloid-beta at much higher levels than human brains do. And drugs which work in mice, lowering brain amyloid and reversing symptoms such as memory loss, have failed to work in people.

As for changing the underlying genes rather than just the protein, science is not yet at this stage for dementia. However, a gene therapy approach is already being trialled in animal models of other neurodegenerative disorders, notably Huntington's.

One alternative would be to go back to using guinea pigs (once so common a model that they passed from scientific to everyday language). They have a human-like *APP* gene. So do dogs and primates, but the ethical tensions, and expense, are much greater for these species.

Burdened brains

A further challenge to the amyloid hypothesis came with the development of neuroimaging methods which could 'see' amyloid plaques in living brains. If too much amyloid-beta is the cause of dementia, you might intuit that more amyloid deposits would mean worse cognition. Yet it soon became apparent that some people with heavy amyloid burdens showed few if any clinical signs of cognitive dysfunction. Post-mortem studies also reported that some brains with plenty of amyloid had belonged to people without signs of dementia. This is why Alzheimer's disease is defined by reference to brain pathology (levels of tau and amyloid-beta), not by the cognitive symptoms used to diagnose dementia. As with other illnesses, like heart disease or cancer, a person can have Alzheimer's without knowing it...for a while.

There are further puzzles. One study found that brain-injured patients with higher amyloid levels had better, not worse, outcomes than those with less of the protein. Also, research on people with dementia and on healthy volunteers suggests that levels of amyloid-beta in CSF are lower, not higher, in patients than in controls—and that levels may begin to drop years before their clinical symptoms become apparent. The strange implication is that a decrease in extracellular amyloid, rather than having too much of it around, could precede—and cause?—Alzheimer's.

These and further criticisms have led some researchers to think (I quote from the leading journal *Nature*) that 'the amyloid hypothesis is dead' and to see further work on it as 'flogging a dead horse'. Most, however, continue to work with some modified version of it. The modifications they advocate are many and various, but can be grouped into three broad types. These can be glossed as: 'more research needed', 'too little too late', and 'more causes needed'.

More research needed

This familiar scientific argument doubles down by saying that the amyloid hypothesis is not yet sophisticated enough. If we knew more about how amyloid-beta works in cells, then we would understand the lack of progress in developing treatments, and be able to develop better ones. Brains are really complicated. That the brain is not the only body part involved in dementia makes the challenge still more difficult.

With respect to failed drugs trials, especially earlier ones, amyloid's proponents have hit back by criticizing the methods: poor selection of participants and inadequate measurements, uncertainty over whether the drugs were even reaching the brain, and so on. In doing so, they highlight the fact that methods are far more important in brain research than many people realize. As well as providing the tools to answer questions, methods also drive how scientists think about their work, and which questions get asked. Having techniques for detecting proteins, for example, prompts researchers to think in terms of proteins and pursue protein-related hypotheses, which can easily be tested. This in turn encourages the development of better methods for dealing with proteins—but not so much for fats or carbohydrates, which may also be important in dementia.

The science of dementia was shaped from its foundation by the fact that Alois Alzheimer and his colleagues used a particular type of cell staining technology and identified particular objects—amyloid plaques—in the brains of people with dementia. The reasoning was simple: this is a visible difference between healthy and unhealthy brains, so perhaps it reflects the cause of the ill-health. The next question was: what are plaques made of? Once that was answered, it led to the amyloid hypothesis, and to research attempts to show causation (e.g. by giving animals amyloid-beta and observing the results), clinical attempts to reduce plaques (in the hope of curing dementia), and technological developments (like PET imaging) to better detect the plaques.

Critics point out the potential gap in the reasoning: just because you see a difference between healthy and unhealthy brains, it does not follow that this particular difference must be causing the problem. It might be a side-effect of some other, neglected difference—let's call it X. To which a proponent of amyloid can then retort: Fine; let's see this neglected difference of yours. Show me that X is really different in the brains of people with Alzheimer's.

Here again methods matter. Perhaps no one has thought of X being involved, or even knows that X exists. Perhaps X has a few devotees seen as cranks by the majority; or perhaps most research attention is simply focused elsewhere. Whatever the reason, X's neglect is likely to be accompanied by less technological sophistication. An example is the use of PET neuroimaging, in which tracers for amyloid were developed and in clinical use some years before tau tracers began to be considered. Thus a new technique may be feasible, but unavailable until enough people take it seriously. Usually that happens because cracks appear in the dominant story, and more researchers start contemplating alternatives. Until then, however, those who seek to prove the importance of X are at a disadvantage.

Too little too late

The second type of explanation as to why the amyloid hypothesis has borne so little clinical fruit (so far) has to do with timing. It argues that Alzheimer's-type neurodegeneration may begin decades before clinical symptoms appear—which is why some people scan positive for amyloid but don't show cognitive dysfunction. For example, there are genetic forms of Alzheimer's in which the age at which the disease begins to bite can be predicted fairly well. Studies of affected families suggest that changes in amyloid-beta biomarkers can be identified up to thirty years earlier. If this is the case, drugs tested on people already diagnosed with the condition (or who have chosen to take part in a trial) are tested too late. They fail because the degenerative process is already far advanced, and irreversible. Like other complex problems from crime and disorder to poor education, from kids' bad behaviour to climate change, neurodegeneration needs to be addressed early.

Scientists hope that if they can identify people who are likely to develop dementia, using biomarkers, and treat them early enough, they may be able to stop the illness taking hold. Studies of amyloid and tau deposits, post-mortem and in living brains, suggest that the proteins can indeed start to aggregate many years before their impact becomes apparent (perhaps in early adulthood, or even younger). Preventing or reversing that aggregation may therefore mean treating people for decades. The hope is that doing so would prevent their dementia from ever developing, and give them better brain health for the rest of their lives.

This may make sense to Alzheimer's researchers, but it is socially problematic. The drugs used will probably have unpleasant side-effects, so persuading people who do not feel ill to take them—perhaps for all their adult lives—will be challenging. We all know how difficult it is to make, and stick with, even minor lifestyle changes with few ill-effects, such as taking vitamin D or doing more exercise. It's thought that only around half of individuals on long-term medication for chronic diseases manage to maintain their regimen. And that is despite having diagnosed medical problems, and a corresponding incentive to take the pills.

Another enormous difficulty is financial. New drugs can cost at least as much as full-time nursing care per year, so unless pharmaceutical funding models are thoroughly reformed, putting everyone at risk of Alzheimer's onto such a long-term regimen would be prohibitively expensive.

More causes needed

The amyloid cascade hypothesis says that too much amyloid-beta—due to over-production, less clearance, or both—is the cause of Alzheimer's-type neurodegeneration. As so often with broad claims, the devil is in the details of interpretation. What exactly does 'the cause of' mean?

One interpretation is that 'the cause' means 'the only cause'. On this 'Amyloid first!' view, too much amyloid-beta would trigger neurodegeneration even in a perfectly healthy brain (if such a thing exists). Moreover, nothing else could do so. This is the simplest interpretation: one protein to rule them all. Genes are fixed 'recipes', laying down the biological law for the environment to obey. Once the amyloid-producing genes are mutated, the fate of their unfortunate possessor is sealed.

It's safe to say that this is not a widely held position. It's too simple, and nothing about amyloid is simple. In people with higher genetic risk of sporadic Alzheimer's, such as *APOE4* carriers, lifestyle seems to influence when, and perhaps whether, they get dementia. Even in familial Alzheimer's, when a dominant gene is inherited and almost certain to cause early-onset illness, it may be possible to delay its onset and progression by living healthily. This suggests that other causes are contributing to how the disease manifests. Amyloid might be the final common pathway, but there is plenty else going on.

Most people with dementia do not have a post-mortem brain analysis, or an amyloid PET scan. Unless everyone does, it is impossible to prove that every case of Alzheimer's disease involves amyloid-beta. However, scientists could disprove that claim by finding patients whose brain amyloid-beta levels were normal throughout life. (Brain scanning techniques have not yet been around for long enough for scientists to follow individuals from childhood until they get, or do not get, dementia.) Unfortunately, such research would be phenomenally lengthy and expensive, requiring the decades-long follow-up of large numbers of people with repeated amyloid scanning and other measures, followed by post-mortem analysis.

Instead, researchers have looked at people who already have 'probable Alzheimer's', to see if any of them show negative amyloid PET scans. Do such cases exist? Yes. However, a negative PET scan does not necessarily mean that a patient's brain amyloid levels are normal, as current tracers can only 'see' larger aggregates. Oligomers might still be present, and some brains with negative scans can still have amyloid-beta deposits (including plaques). There may also be disagreement about how to interpret borderline scans. Even when the brain is available for post-mortem analysis, pathologists, like other people, may come to different conclusions about which disease the person had.

Yet post-mortem analysis remains the most definitive technique for identifying neurodegenerative diseases, so have there been any reports of dementia cases without significant amyloid-beta deposits? Indeed there have; but they may be explained by the presence of other amyloid proteins: tau, alpha-synuclein, TDP-43, and so on. This has led dementia researcher Clifford Jack and colleagues to propose that biomarkers for these various proteins, and more, could be used in a binary way to classify brains as positive ('+', disease indicated) or negative ('–', for disease not found). For example, a healthy brain would be classified as A–/T–/N–, while a case of advanced Alzheimer's would be A+/T+/N+, where A represents an amyloid biomarker (e.g. a PET scan or CSF measurement), T a tau biomarker, and N a biomarker for neurodegeneration (such as an MRI scan indicating tissue loss). When other biomarkers are assessed, for example for alpha-synuclein or vascular disease, extra categories (S, V) could easily be added.

Using biomarkers, rather than relying on traditional disease labels, has its problems. More work is required on standardizing methods between research groups, on pre-mortem testing for proteins beyond amyloid and tau, and on achieving a consensus about which biomarkers to use. However, the attempt to reduce the definitional confusion around dementia is much needed. Clinical diagnoses of 'probable' Alzheimer's and of vascular dementia overlap considerably when it comes to pathology, and cerebrovascular disease can worsen cognitive problems independent of Alzheimer's. Unfortunately (as guidelines published in 2016 point out), definitions of vascular dementia and vascular cognitive impairment are themselves quite variable. DLB, long underdiagnosed, is also an increasingly common finding, and again overlaps considerably with Alzheimer's. Furthermore, a sizeable subset of dementia cases identified as Alzheimer's may actually be a condition called LATE, defined in 2019, which looks clinically similar to Alzheimer's but involves the protein TDP-43. LATE (limbic-predominant age-related TDP-43 encephalopathy) may affect up to half of people over 80. Its pathology is often found alongside signs of Alzheimer's, and when so found it raises the likelihood of the person being diagnosed with dementia. As the authors of the paper defining LATE remark, 'the diseases of aged human brains are complex: multiple comorbid pathologies are the norm, and there is substantial interindividual variation in neuropathological phenotypes' (that is, in what the damage looks like).

Add in the tendency of patients and public to hear 'probable Alzheimer's disease' as 'Alzheimer's', plus the conflation of 'Alzheimer's' with 'dementia', and the confusion over language multiplies. This is why researchers and clinicians carefully distinguish dementia and cognitive impairment from the underlying brain conditions, even if that means people can have Alzheimer's without having dementia.

Long before LATE arrived on the scene, 'Amyloid first!' was already being stretched to include other proteins than amyloid-beta, and other causes too. 'Amyloid first among equals', perhaps? This view is widely held. Stresses on ageing cells mount up, and there seems to be a point beyond which they can no longer maintain themselves. Abnormally aggregating proteins might help to push them towards, or over, that threshold, but so would other factors, from genetic vulnerabilities to lack of exercise. Intracellular errors, when something goes wrong with the internal mechanics of protein management, membrane maintenance, waste disposal, and so on, are another likely factor. Such errors can result from genetic variation, but they also happen more often in older bodies, as the effects of wear and tear, traumas and challenges, accumulate.

On this view, the more hardships a person faces, the more likely they would be to get dementia, and to get it younger. Luckier individuals would be able to sustain their cognition into old age, even with a heavy burden of abnormal protein. As we shall see in Chapter 4, there is support from the science of dementia risk factors for this more complicated idea, which also better reflects the complexities, vulnerabilities, and resilience of brain cells.

Some critics go further—'Amyloid demoted!' They argue that for neurodegeneration, amyloid-beta production is not the prime cause, nor even an early contributor. Instead they see it as a secondary event, a defensive reaction against threats to brain cell viability (or even perhaps a mere by-product of other processes). The analogy often drawn is with an aspect of the body's immune system: its reactions to sick and damaged cells. Just as too strong an immune response to infection can cause potentially lethal septic shock, so as brains age and more damage occurs, the brain's defensiveness might come to do more harm than good.

Figure 8 is a schematic summary of key issues in current dementia science arising from the clinical failure of drugs based on the amyloid cascade hypothesis.

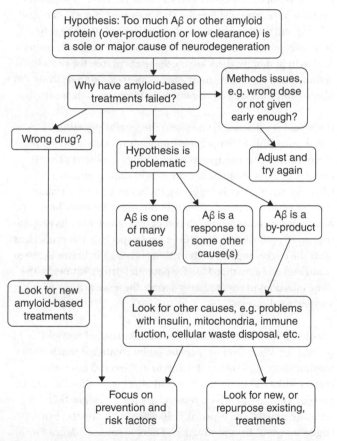

8. The amyloid hypothesis, and beyond (Aβ = amyloid-beta).

As we have seen, the key change required to boost production of amyloid-beta involves favouring beta- over alpha-secretase. The cell can do this, for example, by pulling APP back from the membrane, as stressed cells do. If amyloid-beta production is indeed defensive, increasing its production would be akin to what happens when the immune system detects a problem and activates its cells to respond. As more amyloid-beta is made, its oligomers would accumulate outside cells. They may push already damaged cells beyond the point of survival, or actively kill them (e.g. by puncturing membranes)—again, as happens in immune reactions. And as in immunity, there are mechanisms to stop the process getting out of control. As more oligomers are produced, fibrils and plaques form, soaking up oligomers to damp down their activity.

If amyloid is a defence against neurodegeneration, rather than its initial cause, this has important implications. One is to do with timing. Given that changes in amyloid-beta may start several decades before symptoms of dementia become a problem, whatever other factor is triggering them must happen around then, or earlier. In theory, scientists can use techniques like neuroimaging to decide which comes first, amyloid or its proposed trigger. In practice, this is far from easy, especially if it is not clear what the trigger might be. Many things change in brains between youth and mid-adulthood. As for potential drug treatments, the same questions of cost and long-term adherence arise as with amyloid medications.

Another implication relates to the mechanisms of amyloid processing. We know how genetic faults create too much amyloid-beta, and we are starting to understand how other factors—like APOE proteins—could affect it. But for the 'defence protein' view to be correct, researchers need to show that immune signals, and especially signals of cell damage, can trigger amyloid-beta production. There is some evidence for this. For example, toxic metals like lead are known to stimulate the production of immune chemicals called pro-inflammatory cytokines, and these can stimulate cells to make amyloid-beta. It in turn can trigger production of cytokines and other immune molecules.

There are also implications for treatment. On the 'defence protein' view, treatments based on reducing amyloid are likely to worsen cognition, not improve it. (Some have indeed done so, although that might be via effects on other brain processes.) On the 'by-product' view, amyloid is useful only as a marker of some other, causal process, so treating it is pointless.

Thinking of amyloid-beta as a reaction to other triggers is one way in which researchers are looking beyond the amyloid cascade hypothesis for ideas which could lead to better treatments for Alzheimer's and other forms of dementia. Indeed, the research literature is currently brimming with so many possibilities that the problem is how to choose between them. Finding a potential cause is relatively simple. Finding the causes that lead to successful treatments is much harder.

If not amyloids, what?

Looking beyond misfolded proteins, some potential triggers of neurodegeneration have more support than others. One idea that has moved from the scientific fringe to mainstream thinking has to do with inflammation and immunity.

Most of us can recall a nasty bout of inflammation, whether from an insect bite, flu, or something much more serious like sepsis. Many people suffer from chronic inflammatory and autoimmune diseases like arteriosclerosis or arthritis. Even illnesses traditionally labelled as 'mental', like depression and schizophrenia, are now thought to involve abnormal inflammation. Consequently, medical science has a sizeable array of drugs, already safety-tested, for dealing with it. The hope is that these drugs could be 'repurposed', and used to treat—or at least delay—dementia.

To think about inflammation in dementia, we first need a little background information. The immune system can be divided into two parts: innate and adaptive immunity. Innate immunity evolved first. Its beginnings can be traced back to primitive multicellular organisms—odd though it may be to think of our bodies using the same mechanisms found in sponges and worms. Later, in jawless vertebrates like lampreys, innate immunity began to be supplemented with adaptive immune features. Immune systems, in other words, pre-date brains.

Innate and adaptive immunity protect and serve using both cells and chemicals. Innate immune cells include neutrophils, macrophages, and brain microglia; adaptive immune cells include B and T lymphocytes. Some immune cells are phagocytes (literally 'eater-cells'). Like paramilitary vigilantes, they patrol the body's waterways (blood, lymph, CSF) looking for suspects and dealing out summary justice when they find them. Macrophages, neutrophils, B cells, and the brain's microglia can all act as phagocytes. They detect, then physically consume dangerous material such as viruses, bacteria, and sick or dying cells. T cells meanwhile can lock on to a suspect and bring it to the attention of the nearest phagocyte. Immune cells have other weapons too. They can punch holes in other cells—using mechanisms similar to amyloid pores—or command them to commit suicide.

As long as the identification is correct, immune cells provide an efficient defence. When material is wrongly judged to be hazardous, the body's equivalent of vigilante excess is autoimmune problems.

Immune cells communicate and function by releasing specialized chemical messengers. Some of these are built from fats, but most are proteins. Notable among them are the many kinds of pro- and anti-inflammatory cytokines. These can prompt phagocytes to destroy dangerous material, as well as organizing the removal of damaged tissue and the tidy-up afterwards. Stimulating repair, they also ensure—if they are working properly—that the inflammatory reaction is damped down when it is no longer needed. That wounds can heal, blood vessels and skin cells regrow, and scars fade with time is down to the harmonious interactions of the cytokine choir.

Why have two systems? Innate immunity initially detects and reacts to threats like bacteria and viruses, or physical damage. Its chemicals are the first responders, sounding the alarms which bring phagocytes—rather like phone calls alerting police to a terrorist incident. Some of these chemicals are cytokines, and they serve as signals. Others, like the numerous complement molecules which float through the bloodstream until they bump into a target, can physically bind to unwanted intruders. Like heroic bystanders seizing an attacker so the police can arrest him, they trigger other signals, attracting phagocytes. (Here the analogy breaks down, since police and vigilantes aren't known for eating the people they arrest.)

Bigger crises recruit the slower adaptive immune system. Its cells—B and T lymphocytes—and chemicals—antibodies—bring more powerful, flexible, and targeted responses to particular threats. To do this, they combine fast responses to innate immune signals, rapid genetic mutation, and the ability to clone many copies of themselves very quickly (the cloning happens in lymph glands, which is why these can swell so painfully during infections). The adaptive immune system can also remember an individual's previous encounters with dangerous material. Lots of encounters: it is thought to be capable of recognizing around 100 million distinct hazards, from pollens to pollutants as well as pathogens. Not only can it detect them, but immune memory allows it to deal with them faster and more effectively—and without having to induce the full-scale immune reactions which can leave people at best exhausted, at worst dangerously ill with sepsis. Adaptive immune memory was a crucial evolutionary advance, allowing many familiar infections to be crushed before they could develop into serious threats.

Adaptive immune cells are also important in controlling inflammation, so that it does its healing work without becoming chronic. Abnormalities in adaptive immunity are often found in autoimmune diseases and chronic inflammatory conditions.

Adaptive immunity is why vaccines work. It explains why, when a child brings an infection home from school, not everyone else in the family inevitably gets it; and why repeated infections generally become less severe. It allows people to react to substances, like plastics, to which they were never exposed in our species' long evolutionary history. Adaptive immunity is also the basis of one of the most promising current attempts to treat cancer: immunotherapy, which aims to use the body's own weapons against its rogue cells. The principle is simple: if the immune system can adapt to recognize new threats, perhaps it can be trained to detect and eliminate tumours.

Or, in the case of dementia, abnormal proteins. Exciting current work is looking at ways of using immunotherapy to treat Alzheimer's by altering brain levels of amyloid-beta. To see how this might work, we have to know a little more about neuroimmunology, the study of the brain's immune system.

Fire in the brain

If this book had been written even a decade or two earlier you would have been unlikely to find any mention of the brain's immune system, because it had long been assumed there wasn't one. Instead, scientists thought that the blood–brain barrier kept most bodily hazards at bay. This masterpiece of evolutionary engineering is the layer of cells which separates brain tissue from the network of brain blood vessels: around 400 miles of tubing (the distance from Edinburgh to London or Boston to Washington) crammed into the confines of a human skull.

That tubing is so densely packed that virtually every neuron has its own blood supply. In the tiniest capillaries, which actually deliver the vital nutrients, the walls are only one cell thick, and a slim cell at that. Endothelial cells (the word literally means 'inside-the-nipple', as that was where they were first identified), are fifty times thinner than normal cells: about 0.2 microns, or thousandths of a millimetre. For comparison, the finest silk in the world, Fairy Feather from Japan, is about 150 times thicker, at 30 microns. The total surface area of the blood–brain barrier is thought to be around 20 square metres, about ten times as big as the skin. Yet endothelial cells are so thin that it makes up less than 1 per cent of the brain's total volume. It is a natural wonder, and a highly efficient filter.

When the barrier's efficiency is compromised—for example in brain infections, strokes, or other injuries—researchers assumed that immune cells and chemicals from elsewhere would flood into the brain and deal with the problem. We now know that signals from the damaged brain tissue activate bone marrow, including in the skull, to produce neutrophils. These first-responder phagocytes gather in the damaged area to clear up debris and harmful particles, and signal to recruit adaptive immune cells. In 2018, scientists discovered that neutrophils born in skull marrow can pass through tiny channels in the bone and reach the blood vessels of the meninges, the membranes which wrap and protect the brain. This allows them speedy access to brain tissue.

Unfortunately, invading armies often cause extensive collateral damage, and armies of cytokine-wielding immune cells are no exception. A strong immune response can do a lot of harm to brain tissue. Some areas, such as the hippocampus, are more vulnerable than others. They may be close to areas deep in the brain where the blood–brain barrier is weaker, or they may have receptors for particular immune chemicals which make them more sensitive and easily damaged. (Some of these chemicals also have other functions within the brain, just to complicate matters further.) Whatever the reasons, survivors of brain inflammation are often left with long-term disabilities, like memory problems or impaired motor control. They are also at greater risk for getting dementia.

Brain infections are quite rare, however, as are severe brain damage and stroke. How do brains manage in the less extreme situations they usually have to deal with? We now know that they have their own innate immune cells: microglia.

Microglia are extraordinary cells. Born from stem cells in bone marrow, they take up residence in brain tissue while the foetus is developing, before the blood–brain barrier is formed. They are shape-shifters, able to extend long exploratory tendrils to monitor their environment, or retract into stout rotundity. Like other immune cells, they can also be 'activated' by cytokines and markers of cell damage, which stimulate them to make different sets of proteins—including more immune signals. And they can move within the brain. If a microglial tendril detects a problem, the entire cell can migrate to the site, and if necessary devour the hazardous material.

As this implies, microglia are monitors, signallers, and phagocytes. They emit and respond to an array of chemicals from fellow microglia, from other brain cells like neurons and astrocytes, from the cells of the blood–brain barrier, and from beyond the brain. They defend their neighbours against infections and damage, clear up waste from sick and damaged cells, remove dangerous substances which enter from the bloodstream, and destroy excessive or abnormal proteins. In other words, they work to protect the brain against many of the weaknesses associated with neurodegeneration.

Inflammation in the brain is not quite the same as elsewhere in the body, where it has four 'cardinal signs': redness, swelling, heat, and pain. In a space so constricted, it wouldn't make sense to have swelling; nor are heat and pain experienced when brain tissues are damaged. But the processes, though distinct, serve the same protective functions in brain and body.

This fire is out of control?

Microglia have another role. They prune synapses, in a process involving the innate immune proteins collectively known as complement. Complement can bind to synapses, acting as a tag—an 'eat me' signal—which attracts microglia; these then bite off the synapse. (There is also another innate immune pathway that sends a 'don't eat me' signal to protect more active synapses.) Pruning is essential for healthy brain growth. Humans are born with far more synapses than they need, and lose many of them in the first years after birth. Sometimes this refinement of neural circuitry is deficient, due to problems with innate immune genes (including genes for complement proteins). These problems are linked to developmental disorders such as autism and schizophrenia. Immunity and neurodevelopment, like immunity and neurodegeneration, appear to be tightly interwoven.

Too much pruning later in life could lead to connectivity failures, followed by cell decay and death. This is the pattern of neurodegeneration in dementia; and some researchers think that microglia may be key to understanding it. The idea is that, long before a person is diagnosed, something goes wrong with how their microglia function—and that this, rather than excess amyloid-beta, is the primary trigger of decline.

Phagocytes, including microglia, are usually inactive and quiescent. When a stimulus activates them, however, they can have pro- or anti-inflammatory effects, depending on which cytokine proteins they produce. In a healthy brain, microglial

Beyond amyloid

responses are appropriate to the situation. Microglia age, however, and in ageing brains it seems they can experience the cellular equivalent of burnout through overwork. They become more easily triggered, for longer, and they are more likely to pump out pro-inflammatory than anti-inflammatory cytokines. Thus as we age, the brain's immune environment becomes more inflammation-prone, with more damaging cytokines, and microglia primed to eat synapses and cells.

Just as some people are more likely to suffer from work-related stress, genetic vulnerabilities can make microglia more liable to activation, or less able to do their beneficial work. One of the most significant genetic associations with dementia, after *APOE4*, is a gene for a protein called TREM2. The acronym stands for 'triggering receptor expressed on myeloid 2', and that tells us that TREM2 is a receptor found on myeloid cells (microglia and macrophages) which, when stimulated, activates them. From quietly monitoring, they switch to seek-and-destroy mode. TREM2 helps to control microglial energy levels, and variants linked to Alzheimer's impair its ability to do so. It is also a receptor for amyloid-beta, binding to it and encouraging its removal.

Genetic mutations which affect TREM2 processing are likely to make microglia less able to clear up amyloid-beta. Some such mutations also cause another type of early-onset dementia called Nasu-Hakola disease (NHD). However, NHD is quite different from Alzheimer's, not least in being found mainly in Finland and Japan. In terms of its mental effects, it looks more like early-onset frontotemporal dementia, with social deficits, mood swings, and abnormal, sometimes aggressive behaviour, as well as rapidly progressing cognitive decline. The frontal cortex shows damage to white matter. Physiologically, patients' bones develop large fluid-filled holes and fractures. Fortunately the disease, which typically kills patients before age 50, is extremely rare: at most around two cases per million. (NHD is also known as PLOSL, which stands for an egregious instance of medical jargon: polycystic lipomembranous osteodysplasia with sclerosing leukoencephalopathy.)

There is, in case you were wondering, a TREM1, and it too has implications for dementia. In animal models, a genetic variant which reduces TREM1 production makes microglia less able to eat amyloid-beta, and leads to more amyloid accumulating in the brain.

Research on the role of inflammation in dementia is still in its early stages, and scientists have much more to learn about microglia. However, there is already evidence that raised levels of pro-inflammatory cytokines in ageing, and inflammatory disease, can lead to cellular damage and perhaps neurodegeneration—even when the inflammation starts in the body. Blood-borne cytokines can affect the brain, and many inflammatory conditions, such as diabetes, weaken the blood–brain barrier. Whether inflammation pre-dates, accompanies, or results from amyloid-beta accumulation, and whether it can cause dementia independently of effects on amyloid proteins, is not yet clear. But inflammation is one of the fastest-growing areas of dementia research.

The story so far

Research into dementia in the modern era has been dominated by the amyloid cascade hypothesis. However, while that hypothesis has produced tens of thousands of scientific papers, its clinical outcomes have, to put it mildly, been disappointing. Some commentators criticize this decades-long effort as a huge waste of money and time. Yet to do that is to fail to realize just how complicated a problem researchers face. There are some brain diseases which may be traced to a single defective gene, for which a quick fix will someday be available. With recent advances in genetics, that day could come sooner than we think. But most of the disorders which affect our brains are more like death by a thousand cuts than by a single bullet. If neurodegeneration were simple, it would have been cured by now.

This complexity has left room for other ways of thinking about dementia to develop alongside the biomedical approach: alternatives such as person-centred care and the disability/human rights movement that prioritize the individual rather than the illness. It has also forced scientists to discover a good deal more about human brains, in sickness and in health, than the pioneers who began the field could have imagined would be necessary. In doing so they have learned about much more than Alzheimer's, frontotemporal dementia, DLB, or vascular dementia. We all age, and our brain function changes as we do so, whether or not that change slips into cognitive decline. Understanding how brains age, and which factors make that ageing more or less successful, has implications for every human being. Accepting that many factors contribute to dementia—natural effects of ageing, genetic vulnerabilities, other diseases, traumatic life events—additionally reminds us that this is an illness whose presentation, at least in its earlier stages, is likely to vary considerably, both from day to day and between people. Every brain, life history, and person is unique.

Considering other contributing factors than amyloid also opens up the possibility of new treatments. Looking at inflammation, for example, may allow a formidable array of existing drugs to be re-applied, at much less cost than developing new ones from scratch. Among the candidates are some with promising, if preliminary, signs of clinical benefit.

Treatments, however, are a last resort, especially for illnesses which may smoulder in brain tissue for decades before becoming apparent. And treatments are costly. Alongside clinical research, therefore, many scientists, health economists, and governments favour trying to prevent, or delay, the onset of dementia. Pushing back the start of cognitive decline by even a year would mean fewer people needing expensive drugs, or care, for less time. Ideally, the kind of behaviours which help to prevent dementia would be taught in schools and encouraged in adulthood, making brain health as much of a lifelong habit as maintaining a healthy body weight.

To achieve this, we need to know which behaviours are good, and which bad, for brain health. That brings us to the science of risk factors, our next topic.

Chapter 4
Risk factors

This chapter looks at some of the most hopeful aspects of dementia science: the growing understanding of what makes it more (or less) likely to afflict a person. Can we change our lives to make it less likely to happen to us? The idea is that even quite small lifestyle and social changes could delay the onset of dementia in individuals, reducing the number of people who experience it.

This is not just wishful thinking. With dementia being more often talked about, and more older people around, there is a widespread perception that rates of dementia are rising. Not so. Studies and reviews looking at changes in its prevalence (how common it is), incidence (how many people get it), or mortality (how many people die with it) are finding clear evidence that older populations today are less affected by dementia than in previous decades. Yes, more people are living longer, but in general they are doing so with fewer years of cognitive impairment and severe ill-health. Something has changed—at least in Western Europe and the USA. Research carried out elsewhere has found varying trends: for instance, rising dementia prevalence in Japan, low prevalence in India, stable incidence in Nigeria, large regional differences in China.

A tentative science

Why might this be? To understand more about why rates of dementia are changing, we need to think about what factors might raise the risk of dementia, or decrease it. That is the domain of epidemiology. The word relates to epidemics: diseases that act upon (epi) the people (demos). Epidemiologists generally work with very large, sometimes nationally representative samples, looking for patterns of association between the presence of disease and potential risk (or protective) factors. Epidemiology is one of the more widely misunderstood scientific methods, so before we look at the epidemiology of dementia, it's worth briefly reviewing the overall approach.

Epidemiology can be a very expensive exercise, involving the creation and maintenance of healthcare databases, the scouring of previous literature for meta-analyses, and/or the recruitment and study of thousands of participants. (That is for studies within a single country; cross-cultural research is even more demanding.) For slow, insidious illnesses like dementia, such studies can take years to get results. Identifying trends through time is even more challenging, requiring long-term comparisons that use the same or similar methods, perhaps over decades. This is particularly difficult when definitions and ways of assessing the disease, or potentially relevant environmental and social factors, have changed; or when different research groups are defining risks and diseases differently—as has frequently been the case for dementia.

Epidemiologists look for patterns of association: statistical probabilities, not guarantees. Correlations—associations between a risk factor (R) and a disease (D)—are much easier to find than proof that R causes D. Ice cream consumption is correlated with drowning because on hot days more people eat ice cream and more go swimming, not because ice cream causes drowning.

The correlation could still show up in the statistics even if not a single person both ate an ice cream and then drowned.

Moreover, epidemiology looks at groups; it does not directly address individual risk. When a news headline reports that, for example, eating processed meat doubles the risk of getting diabetes, the implication is that the risk applies to you, the reader. Which it may, if you are similar in all relevant respects to the people from whom the statistic was derived. If most research is done on white Western students, or males, or adults, the results may still apply to other groups in other countries; but they may not. The best research takes samples which reflect the population from which they are drawn—and reports results accordingly. Inferring grand claims about humanity based on a convenient pool of students and work colleagues is no longer the scientific norm it used to be.

Incidentally, a claim like 'doubles the risk' is unhelpful alarmism unless you know what number is being doubled—the baseline rate. Having twice the chance of getting a disease that only affects one in every hundred thousand (0.001 per cent) is not likely to be a big concern. If the risk is one in ten (10 per cent), however…maybe it's time to think about that lifestyle change? Bear in mind too that statistics often refer to lifetime risk, and that will vary with how much life the person's had. For example, a large 2018 study of neurological disease risks found that the risk of developing dementia, stroke, or Parkinson's disease was 48 per cent (almost one in two) in women and 36 per cent (roughly one in three) in men—when those men and women were aged 45. For other ages, the percentages would be different.

There are other pitfalls. With such large numbers, care must be taken that apparently significant results are not mere statistical flukes. As with the ice cream/drowning example (where a third factor, temperature, is the underlying cause), there is also the question of 'what else might explain this?' Take too many factors into account, and the study will become unfeasibly large. Too few, and some crucial factor could be overlooked.

Asking what was not done is often informative. For example, immense amounts of animal research have been carried out, and conclusions drawn about human brains and behaviour, on male animals only. It's quicker and cheaper, since it halves the numbers needed. But the conclusions drawn affect women as well as men. (The traditional justification for this bias was that variation in female hormones made interpreting data too difficult. Yet recent studies—recent because it took so long to notice the problem—find that male hormones also vary. Indeed, they fluctuate as much if not more than females', and less predictably.)

Any human study must also be wary of selection bias: could the findings have been influenced by the choice of participants? For example, researching the effects of poverty and time pressure on cognitive function using volunteer participants (who tend to be middle-class and to have time to help with research) might not be the best strategy. With illnesses like dementia, there is also the issue of survivor bias to consider. Could those volunteers who are well enough to take part, or still alive by the end, be different in some relevant way from those who aren't—and might this influence the results?

Scientists being neither gods nor robots, experimenter bias may also have a role, especially when dealing with human patients. Are some participants treated differently by the researchers, consciously or unconsciously? Could the experimenter's body language be giving too much away? (This is why drug trials are double-blinded, so that neither the participant nor the experimenter knows who is getting the drug and who the placebo.)

Even if all these traps for heffalumps are avoided, as they can be with careful research design, research needs to be reproduced before it can be fully trusted. (This is why the discussion sections of research papers are littered with words such as 'potential', 'possible', and 'may'.)

Science and the media

Yet it's remarkable how a hesitant scientific conclusion can firm up by the time it finds itself installed in a headline or a press release. In science, certainty is, or should be, a signal to proceed with caution. Scientists learn to think in terms of more accurate approximations to reality, leaving absolute truths to religion. In the media, however, certainty is more like a prerequisite. It emerges naturally from the compression of language used in headlines—the sections of news most widely consumed and most likely to be remembered. Under intense competition, strong messages are considered more appealing to busy readers.

Such firming up can leave news consumers confused as to how seriously to take the latest health scare or breakthrough. When new science is reported with undue conviction, its caveats lost, and its uncertainty downplayed, later work which reduces this uncertainty may not be reported at all; or it may be presented in adversarial terms, as a correction or contradiction. This leaves people convinced, incorrectly, that scientists continually flip-flop and haven't a clue. The problem is not limited to epidemiology. It also applies to other research relevant to dementia, from neuroscience and psychology to medicine and biochemistry.

Public reports of risk factor science, however, are especially vulnerable to a more subtle cognitive trap than the lure of certainty: the myth of perfection. Media accounts often seem to imply that a perfect lifestyle is a real possibility. If only you would regulate your existence properly, you would be able to enjoy good health of body and mind until you expired. Poor health, it follows, must be your personal responsibility. Either you deliberately sinned, or you failed to follow good advice, or you didn't learn how best to look after yourself until it was too late. Advertising carries the same assumptions, but with an easier offer on how to improve your lifestyle, provided you can afford to buy the product.

I trust that by caricaturing this myth so bluntly I have exposed its status as pernicious nonsense. Victim-blaming is a dangerous human habit. It is cruel, and it neglects an enormous amount of scientific evidence, as well as common sense. We are not, and cannot be, entirely responsible for our physical or our mental health. Not only did we not select our parents, our genes, or our childhood environments, but we are constantly being affected by factors beyond our control—sometimes even beyond our power to detect. Which kind of death you will have, and which illnesses will haunt you prior to death, has much more to do with luck than with any failings of willpower and self-control. You may live an exemplary lifestyle, and still end it in the shadows of dementia. Or you may pursue the kind of life which gives healthcare professionals palpitations, and yet be granted your vision of a good death. Accurately predicting one individual's fate is rarely possible.

Nevertheless, it is worth paying attention to probabilities. Many people who thought dementia wouldn't happen to them went on to live and die with the condition. As with smoking and cancer, we may be able to think of someone who did beat the odds despite a high-risk lifestyle—especially when we are contemplating the effort of making changes to our own habits. But memory is a motivated process, biased by what we want to believe. Most of us do not beat the odds.

Types of risks

Despite the caveats surrounding epidemiology, there is now plenty of research on risk factors for dementia. To explore it, we can begin by grouping them into three types. One is the genetic lottery: does the person have a *PSEN* mutation, or one or two copies of the *APOE4* allele, or of the many other genes thought to raise dementia risk by small amounts? The second type of risk is environmental: external factors such as poverty or pollution that affect people's chances of getting dementia. (Here, 'environmental' includes both biological factors that primarily affect the brain via the body, like smoking or chemotherapy, and social/psychological factors working via the mind, which can be as powerful as childhood abuse or as subtle as the long-term build-up of beliefs about dementia.) The third type of risk, linking nature and nurture, is physiological: aspects of how the body works, or doesn't work, which affect the function and structure of the brain.

Chapter 2 looked at the major genetic risk factors for dementia, so this chapter will focus on physiological and environmental factors. These are inextricably linked, not least because most environmental factors affect the brain indirectly, by changing the body's physiology (radiation damage is an exception). Physiological risks depend on the person's genes, their current environment, and their life history, including, we now know, pre-birth and perhaps even pre-conception events.

Two key concepts underpin any discussion of risk factors. The first is whether the risk is modifiable. Traditionally, 'nature' and genes were identified with fixed, unchangeable influences, while 'nurture' and the environment were considered more malleable. Even before scientists found ways to manipulate genes directly, however, that idea of fixed-versus-fluid was simplistic. For one thing, it depends on drawing a clear distinction between genetic and other factors. One example is biological sex, usually assigned as male (XY chromosomes) or female (XX chromosomes). Yet even genetically defined sex (let alone gender) is more variable than this dichotomy suggests. One can, for instance, have XXY chromosomes. One can also have reassignment surgery.

Sex and gender are very relevant to our topic, not least because women are more likely to experience dementia. Why? Part of the reason is that they tend to live longer. When that is taken into account, however, it is not yet clear how much of the remaining difference is down to factors relating to biological sex and how much to gender-related cultural factors. Long-term follow-up studies of people who go through gender reassignment might help to answer these questions, but such research has not yet been done.

Moreover, with the discovery of epigenetics it became apparent that cells can 'dial up' (or down) the activity of their genes, changing the amount of protein they produce, and hence their effects. Chemical tags are constantly being applied to, or removed from, DNA by a sophisticated array of cellular enzymes, and these tags tell the genetic machinery to make more or less RNA and protein. Thus although the list of genes you got from your parents is fixed, how those genes are used can vary in response to changes in the cell's environment, including chemicals in the diet, hormones, and signals from neighbouring cells. This is why what you eat and drink, how much exercise you take, and even how you appraise a situation can permanently alter your body and brain. 'Genetic' does not mean 'set in stone'.

Just as genetic influences are less fixed than they may seem, so many environmental risks which are in theory preventable are not actually prevented. Some of these, such as childhood trauma, can have lifelong, tremendously damaging impacts on a person. Yet although it is horribly easy for someone to abuse a child, it is extremely difficult to mitigate the harm. In other words, a supposedly malleable effect, once it has happened, may not look so malleable. The time at which such impacts happen during a life is also crucial.

A further point, as obvious and yet frequently overlooked, is that many environmental effects cannot be changed by individuals. You probably have less control than you would like over where you live, which cultural hang-ups you inherited, what you spend your time doing, how healthy and wealthy your neighbours are, and how stressed or secure you feel—and the poorer you are, the less control you have. You have little control over how climate change is affecting your locality, or what poisons you are breathing or eating. And you have no control over many events, like earthquakes or terrorist atrocities, which can seriously affect your mental and physical environment.

The second key concept, which interacts with the first, is that of reverse causation (see Box 1). Many supposed risk factors for dementia may in fact themselves be caused by the disease taking hold. Late-life anxiety, depression, or weight loss, for example, might all precede a diagnosis of dementia, but that does not

Box 1 Reverse causation

Normally we think of a risk factor R (e.g. smoking or brain infection) causing a disease D (e.g. lung cancer, dementia)—if not guaranteeing the disease, at least making it more likely. But what if cause and effect are the other way round, such that D is causing R?

For example, earlier retirements, less intellectually demanding careers, and lack of hobbies have all been linked to a greater chance of developing dementia. This could be because the lack of stimulation leads to unused synapses withering away. The risk factor of mental inactivity would cause neurodegeneration to set in, facilitating dementia. Use it or lose it. R causes D.

Yet there could be another explanation. Dementia diagnoses are usually preceded by a long, slow accumulation of cognitive difficulties. These might be forcing people to retire earlier, switch to less effortful careers, or cut down on other activities. This would be reverse causation: D causing R. Reverse causation is more likely when the supposed risk R is measured shortly before the disease D is recognized, and in conditions with a long, slow build-up, like dementia.

necessarily mean they are causing the cognitive impairment. Instead, neurodegenerative changes might already be affecting brain areas that regulate metabolism or mood, generating symptoms not yet recognized as such. Plus, cognitive symptoms due to neurodegeneration might also be contributing, for instance by leading the person to forget meals, or to worry about their forgetfulness.

Disentangling the webs of cause and effect is crucial, because scientists are looking for modifiable risk factors. Depression due to, say, loneliness, or even depression in reaction to a feared illness, might be treatable. But if the depression has an organic basis—neurodegeneration—then this supposedly modifiable risk factor may not be modifiable after all.

Bearing in mind these caveats, let us look at some of the major risk factors for dementia.

Age

One risk factor beyond our grasp is the passage of time, so age would seem to be firmly in the 'non-modifiable' category. Unfortunately, getting older is also the biggest risk factor for dementia, as it is for disease in general. Alzheimer's Disease International (ADI)—an organization which draws together national dementia societies such as the Alzheimer's Society (UK), the Alzheimer's & Related Disorders Society of India, Foundation Alzrus (Russia), and the Alzheimer's Association (USA)—has estimated that, across the world, nearly 10 million people acquire the condition every year. (By 2050, more than 150 million are likely to have it.) As more people live longer, thanks to advances in public health and medicine, they—we—become more likely to experience dementia.

The 2016 Global Burden of Disease study for Alzheimer's and dementia found that estimates of dementia prevalence ranged from around 0.4 per cent in Nigeria and Ghana to almost three times as high in Turkey (bearing in mind that diagnostic and data-collection procedures vary greatly across countries). Those are overall figures, as prevalence rises rapidly after age 60. In the UK, among people aged 60–64 the prevalence of dementia is reckoned at just under one in a hundred (0.9 per cent). How it changes beyond that age is shown in Figure 9 for men (solid black line) and women (grey dashed line). By age 65–69 the prevalence has nearly doubled, to 1.7 per cent; by age 75–79 that figure has

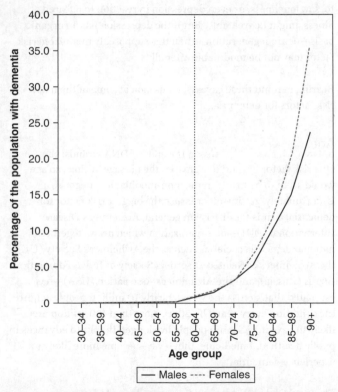

9. Dementia prevalence in the UK. Prevalence rises sharply at older ages.

more than tripled to 6 per cent; by 85–89 it has tripled again, to 18.3 per cent. Among people aged 95 or older, more than four in every ten have dementia (41.1 per cent). Of course, even in the rapidly ageing UK few people reach this age.

Yet the risks that time brings are not shared out equally. We know, and science has confirmed, that people age at different rates, depending on both their genes and the environmental stresses they face during life. Two people with the same chronological age may have different biological ages, and hence different risks of premature death and ageing-related diseases. Social traumas, like abuse, and biological stresses, like malnutrition, also seem to accelerate cell ageing. For health problems, the Matthew effect is noticeable: to them that already have troubles, more will be given.

Biological age can be measured in a number of ways, such as counting the number of epigenetic tags on DNA (the 'epigenetic clock'), looking at bone growth, or measuring the length of tiny structures called telomeres in blood cells. (Telomeres are segments of DNA which sit like caps on the ends of DNA strands; they seem to shorten with age.) Scientists are still working out which method, or combination of methods, is best; this is a very new field. What is clearer is that it is biological, not chronological, age which is the risk factor for dementia. And although we can't change time, biological age might be more malleable.

Delaying biological ageing has been a human dream for centuries, but only now do we have the tools to understand the problem and its potential solutions. One long-standing idea involves changing metabolism. Innumerable flies, worms, and rodents have starved for science to demonstrate that caloric restriction (cutting calories by up to 40 per cent) has benefits for health and longevity in these species. Unfortunately, human volunteers find caloric restriction extremely difficult to do, and especially to keep doing, and there is relatively little research on its long-term effects. Yet intensive study of the many changes which come with getting older, alongside better understanding of epigenetics and cell biology, has encouraged a renewed scientific focus on food restriction and other ways to 'treat' ageing.

Many cell processes work less well as time passes, from the mitochondria supplying our cells with energy to the immune system that protects us from infections. Research into why this happens still has far to go, but many scientists point to environmental damage: from toxic chemicals, ultraviolet radiation, and so on. For example, components of junk food and polluted air can stimulate inflammation and damage cell membranes, while UV can disrupt DNA. (Severe problems with DNA repair are found in rare but terrible diseases like Cockayne syndrome, in which ageing appears to be drastically speeded up.) Damage to cell enzymes, membranes, and genetic material is part of the wear and tear of everyday life, and in young, healthy cells it is kept in check by efficient maintenance processes. With ageing, however, these processes themselves can be disrupted.

One of the foremost means by which the wear and tear of ageing is actually inflicted on the body—and the brain—is oxidative stress. We need oxygen to live, but it is a dangerous material, easily forming molecules called free radicals. These can seriously damage cells (indeed, the immune system uses them to kill bacteria). They can interfere with mitochondria and weaken or puncture cell membranes. This is a particularly severe problem for neurons because—with their long axons and extensive dendrites—they have so much membrane to maintain. Free radicals can prevent proteins from folding properly, disrupting many cell systems. And they can cause epigenetic changes which lead to inaccurate read-outs of DNA and RNA. Eventually, cell function becomes so impaired that it is unsustainable: death by a thousand chemical reactions.

(Fear of oxidative stress is why many people take antioxidant supplements, though evidence for their effectiveness is inconclusive. Eating lots of fresh fruit and vegetables as an anti-ageing strategy has more research support.)

Wear and tear may also contribute to the body's tendency to produce less of certain beneficial chemicals as it gets older. Among these are growth-stimulating blood factors; and this has led some scientists to experiment with a technique called parabiosis, in which a young animal's blood supply is linked to that of an old animal to achieve rejuvenation. (In humans, the equivalent process would be blood transfusions; when the research was published this led to excited headlines about vampire seniors.) Work is ongoing to identify the specific factors responsible for improving the older animals' health. Perhaps one day a simple injection might keep us young, with blood transfusions saved for emergencies. Perhaps.

Another challenge of ageing is that the body's ability to renew its cells is limited. Most can divide to produce daughter cells up to about fifty times—the best-known exceptions are cancer cells, which can go on dividing indefinitely. In a young, healthy person, sick cells destroy themselves, or send signals instructing immune cells to destroy them. In older or less healthy individuals, however, they may either turn cancerous or switch into a diseased state called senescence, in which they pump out harmful molecules. Studies in animals which attempted to clear out senescent cells from organs using 'senolytic' drugs have found beneficial effects on ageing, and pronounced cellular senescence has been found in the brains of people with Alzheimer's. Genetic faults affecting programmed cell suicide have also been linked to dementia. Cell senescence is now a hot topic in the race to develop anti-ageing drugs.

Slowing the clock

Biological ageing is the biggest risk factor for dementia, but it is a surprisingly modifiable risk factor. There is much we can do to lower the toll that passing years inflict upon our bodies. We know this, because it is already being done. Scientists are fairly sure that the reason dementia rates are falling in Western countries, and perhaps elsewhere, is that several major causes of unhealthy ageing have also decreased in the past half-century. Toxins such as lead, which is known to damage brains and impair cognition, have been reduced. Nutrition has improved, the rise in obesity notwithstanding. Better housing and infrastructure have arguably helped lower social stresses like noise pollution as well as physical ones like infectious disease. And the number of people getting prolonged education, which is associated with a lower risk of dementia, is much higher these days.

There have been other changes too. In the UK, for example, adult smoking rates have dropped from nearly half the post-war population to less than a sixth in 2017. Levels of air pollution have also fallen in Western and other countries. Both smoking and pollution are known risks for dementia. Both cause oxidative stress and damage to the heart, lungs, and blood vessels. In animal experiments, realistic levels of pollution increase brain deposits of amyloid-beta. In humans, long-term exposure has been found to result in worse cognitive performance (e.g. on tests of verbal ability), an effect which is more pronounced among older people. The particulates in car exhausts, which include carbon, sodium, and ammonium particles, are thought to be especially damaging, since some are so tiny that they can get into the brain and cause an inflammatory reaction. Particulate levels are now falling in a majority of countries, as public awareness of their dangers grows.

The percentage of people drinking alcohol has also fallen by about 5 per cent, worldwide, since the year 2000. There is regional variation, with reductions in Europe and Africa and a rise in China. (Bear in mind these regions' very different histories with alcohol. Europeans have been swigging it for generations; consumption in Muslim nations tends to be low; and consumption in China, though rising, is lower than in the West.)

In Europe and the Americas, binge drinking, which does the most harm to body and brain, has been falling for decades.

There are many pathways to cell damage and decline, and many risk factors influence the likelihood of getting dementia. The search for a causal 'Factor X', a target for modification, faces an overwhelming number of candidates. However, there is a simpler way of looking at the problem of dementia risk: in terms of overall health. Poor health, both mental and physical, raises the chance of cognitive decline. Vascular, lung, and kidney disease, poverty and chronic stress, alcohol dependence and abuse, smoking and pollution, poor diet, and more—these factors bias human brains towards mental illness, physical diseases, and cognitive impairment. Thus preventing and treating ill-health should lead to fewer people with dementia.

Again, there is already evidence for this approach. Falling dementia rates in Western countries have been accompanied, and most likely preceded, by improvements in welfare and public healthcare (some of which however have stalled in recent years, under the pressure of financial austerity). Better treatments for stroke, heart disease, and traumatic brain injury have reduced their impact on long-term cognitive function. Screening for and treating high blood pressure, high cholesterol, and diabetes has also led to reductions in cardiovascular and cerebrovascular disease (including stroke); these are major risk factors for dementia. The hope is that this approach, which seems to be working in the West, will work worldwide. Only a third of people with dementia live in high-income countries, so even just extending screening programmes globally could greatly reduce the incidence of cognitive—and other—problems.

Blood and brain

Healthy blood and its efficient transportation to brain cells are critically important. The brain is a hungry organ, taking around a quarter of the body's energy; when blood flow is cut off, unconsciousness and death rapidly follow. The blood–brain barrier protects neurons and glia by filtering out poisons, while allowing in oxygen, glucose, and other nutrients. It also lets in chemical signals which tell the brain how well the body is working, whether there is infection present, when the person last ate, and much else besides.

Unfortunately, both blood vessels and the blood–brain barrier become more vulnerable as we age. In a stroke, large blood vessels like the cerebral arteries can tear (haemorrhagic stroke) or block up (ischaemic stroke). Stroke is a major cause of death and disability, and having one can double the risk of dementia. The WHO estimates that in 2016, strokes killed nearly six million people a year, making them the second biggest cause of death after heart disease. That said, rates of stroke, like those of heart disease, have been falling for over a century (and more quickly since the 1970s) in Western countries.

As we grow older, our hearts tend to beat less efficiently. As cardiac function falls with age, brain blood flow slows, delivering nutrients and removing waste less efficiently. What's good for the heart is therefore good for the brain, as a healthy heart promotes strong cerebral blood flow. Exercise, which helps the heart to work better, is thought to be one of the best ways of protecting ageing brains.

Yet even before blood flow problems come to doctors' notice, older brains develop tiny holes where miniature strokes have damaged the blood–brain barrier. As these accumulate they start to affect cognitive function. When detected with MRI scans or in post-mortem studies, they are labelled as 'small vessel disease', a precursor to vascular dementia.

Most strokes are due to brain blockages. These are often imagined as miniature fatbergs, built from the same materials that clog up arteries elsewhere in the body: mostly fats, including cholesterol. This is why dietary advice has for years emphasized the importance of reducing fat intake, and particularly the intake of saturated and trans-fats, as well as the importance of keeping blood cholesterol levels low. So far, the scientific jury is out on whether taking statins to lower cholesterol protects against dementia. Since most people put on statins are of an age where neurodegeneration might be setting in anyway, it is proving hard to rule out reverse causation. For example, patients already showing cognitive impairment might be less likely to be prescribed statins, and more likely to forget to take them.

Some brain blockages, however, are mostly made of proteins, notably our old acquaintance amyloid-beta. In ageing brains it can build up on vessel walls, stifling blood flow, causing toxins to build up, and strangling the life out of nearby cells. Such damage is extensive in vascular dementia but is also found in Alzheimer's and other types.

Damage to blood vessels, furthermore, reduces the supply of oxygen to the brain (causing hypoxia). This can stress brain cells, and in extreme cases destroy them. Certain areas, like the hippocampus and hypothalamus, are particularly vulnerable. Severe acute oxygen shortages, or chronically underperforming oxygen delivery, can facilitate later cognitive dysfunction, as well as worsening metabolic problems like insulin resistance. Unsurprisingly, hypoxia at birth, sleep apnoea (disturbed breathing at night, often due to obesity), and lung diseases such as COPD have all been linked to an increased risk of dementia.

Blood sugar problems

High cholesterol and high blood pressure are not the only conditions that can damage blood vessels and the brain cells that depend on them. Another common risk factor for dementia, and a big public health concern in its own right, is diabetes. Extremes of either high or low blood sugar (hyper- or hypoglycaemia), and, especially, rapid swings between the two, stress brain cells and can weaken the blood–brain barrier. Such swings are characteristic of diabetes and its precursor, insulin resistance. Untreated, they may raise the risk of cognitive decline and dementia by around 50 per cent.

In diabetes the pancreas, which normally produces insulin, malfunctions. Often this is due to poor diet and lack of exercise; but although obese people are at higher risk of diabetes, lifestyle choices are by no means the whole story. There are many diabetics who are not obese—former UK prime minister Theresa May is a well-known example—and there are several varieties of diabetes. Genes, autoimmune disease, severe physical traumas like chemotherapy, and ageing can all play a role. So can environmental stresses like air pollution, sleep deprivation and shift work, chronic stress, and poverty. We still have much to learn about diabetes.

As insulin production fails, cells have trouble getting the nutrients they need. This can lead to vascular damage, cell death, and eventually the serious complications of diabetes: heart disease, blindness, amputation, kidney failure, and so on. Nutrient supply problems also contribute to brain dysfunction, but insulin there does more than regulate blood sugar. It helps control metabolism by acting on the hypothalamus. It is also good for neuronal and synaptic growth. And it protects against cell damage, making it a potential treatment for dementia. Insulin treatments are already being tested for cognitive dysfunction.

Diabetes may not be fully understood, but it has a range of treatments available (not least exercise, which shares many of insulin's beneficial effects). Indeed, better identification and management of diabetes may be one of the reasons why dementia rates are falling. Taking the common diabetes drug metformin long-term, for instance, has been linked to better late-life cognition. Untreated diabetes is a severe health hazard, but the risks are much reduced if the illness is well managed.

Of course, it would be preferable if people could avoid getting diabetes, and other illnesses which raise the risk of dementia, in the first place. Sometimes this isn't possible—if the pancreas is damaged by autoimmune disease, for instance—but even then exercise and eating healthily are unlikely to hurt, and may well help, the patient. Improved control of blood sugar levels is only one benefit of a healthy lifestyle. Eating well, for example, can boost brain resilience in other ways too, from providing essential micronutrients to reducing the build-up of damage to blood vessels. And accumulating evidence from long-term prospective studies (where scientists take a group of people and watch to see what happens) suggests that some diets are much better for brain resilience than others. The healthiest are those, like the Mediterranean diet, which include more fruit and veg, nuts, wholegrains, and fish, and less meat, sugar, and heavily processed food. The least healthy are high in fat, salt, sugar, and chemical additives, but low in fibre, and in micronutrients such as the omega-3 fatty acids and B-vitamins.

Inflammation

Eating well, taking exercise, and other features of a healthy lifestyle (e.g. good sleep) may also help to keep the immune system working well, reducing the impact of infections and toxins and the damaging effects of inflammation. Acute inflammatory reactions to microbes in the body are often minor inconveniences, but they can be devastating. When pathogens get into brain tissue, the inflammatory response can lead to encephalitis, which can be lethal. Bacterial meningitis kills around a tenth of people it infects, and many survivors experience cognitive problems, for example with memory. Encephalitis also raises the risk of cognitive impairment later in life.

Yet other infections can also affect cognition, even without themselves reaching the brain. We all know the 'brain fog' that comes with flu or norovirus. Caregivers for people with pre-existing cognitive impairment often observe that even a mild respiratory infection can exacerbate symptoms. The culprits in both cases are thought to be pro-inflammatory cytokines, either slipping through the blood–brain barrier or produced by brain cells themselves. Moreover, inflammation is an acute response to infection; but it can become chronic, as in obesity, stress, or autoimmune conditions like arthritis. That prolonged exposure to cytokines, though less intense than in acute inflammation, can still harm brain cells.

Unsurprisingly, many factors thought to raise the risk for dementia involve inflammation. Among them are pollution, smoking, poor diet, poor dental and oral health, sleep loss, physical inactivity, infections, and inflammatory diseases. (Many of these are modifiable, though with some—such as oral health and inactivity—reverse causation may be relevant.) The list also includes major surgery, which has been linked to cognitive decline, especially in elderly patients and when general anaesthetics are involved.

In addition, concussion and traumatic brain injury (TBI), with and without loss of consciousness, are likewise increasingly recognized as dangerous. In the UK, researchers are beginning to study the effects of repeatedly heading the ball on footballers' brains. In the USA, military research is tackling the problem of brain injury caused by improvised explosive devices. Concerns about boxing have been around for decades; concerns about other contact sports, like rugby and American football, are growing. (Even quite easily modifiable risk factors must be not only recognized but taken seriously, and the inertia of the status quo overcome, before people make the necessary changes.) Yet the biggest cause of TBI is not sporting or combat injuries, but having a fall, followed by traffic accidents.

Lack of use

Inflammation, and other damaging processes like oxidative stress, affect brain cells in numerous ways. Among their earliest targets in ageing, and much more so in dementia, are the synapses neurons use to communicate. Complement proteins, boosted in inflammatory reactions, are involved in synaptic pruning, and certain cytokines alter synaptic plasticity and learning. Oxidative stress impairs both synaptic membranes and the intricate mechanisms by which neurotransmitters are shuttled to the surface, released, and then recycled. As noted in Chapter 1, synapses are thought to be among the first casualties of neurodegeneration. When they die, brain cells can become unviable.

Many of the genes implicated in Alzheimer's affect how synapses work. Each variant by itself has a small effect on disease risk—much smaller than the *APOE* gene—but they add up to a pattern of vulnerability or resilience. This inheritance makes each individual brain more or less susceptible to connection failures, and more so as the brain gets older. However, life events can also affect how these genes behave—how much protein they produce, where, and when—and hence how well the brain's connections work.

In a flourishing neighbourhood, people talk to each other, and the same is true for brain cells. As well as adequate supplies and efficient waste disposal, this requires healthy synapses, and healthy axons to carry neural messages over long distances. It also needs the community to be diverse, as the various kinds of glial cells are crucial for brain function. And to thrive, brain cells need to use their communicative talents: to be actively connected with their fellows. (Again, the human analogy presents itself.) That requires them to be stimulated, ultimately by sensory inputs from the eyes, ears, and elsewhere. With the brain, as with muscle strength, 'use it or lose it' seems to be the rule. Cognitive risk factors for dementia, therefore, should have in common the reduction of brain stimulation, and indeed, this appears to be the case (albeit bearing in mind reverse causation).

For example, sensory failings, such as a poor sense of smell and hearing loss, are frequently found in people at high risk of dementia. Physical inactivity also reduces brain inputs, from the many sensors in our muscles as well as from the changing environments through which we move. This is one reason why exercising by way of a walk in the park may be more beneficial than walking on a treadmill in the gym: the environment is richer.

Brain stimulation, however, goes beyond these inputs, important though they are. One of the more consistent, and consistently puzzling, findings in dementia research is that education and lifelong learning are protective. Highly educated people still get dementia, but they tend to get it later, and when it is finally diagnosed the decline may be faster. It is as if the habit of thinking tops up a cognitive reserve, allowing people to withstand the effects of neurodegeneration for longer (as well as helping to stave off boredom).

Cognitive reserve is related to but distinct from brain reserve, the capacity to keep going despite considerable loss of synapses, neurons, and glia. Brains have a limited ability to grow new cells, but they are immensely flexible and resilient: able to reroute their circuits, alter neurotransmitter production, repair damage to some extent, or recruit new areas to compensate. In dementia, symptoms begin long after neurodegeneration. In multiple sclerosis, symptoms can be intermittent ('relapsing-remitting MS') for up to twenty years before the condition starts getting progressively worse. The motor symptoms used to diagnose Parkinson's, such as tremor, may only appear after up to half the substantia nigra's cells have died. All this is only possible because of the brain's capacity to reorganize its functions after damage.

The relationships between physical and mental resilience—between brain reserve and cognitive reserve—are not yet fully understood. Nor is it clear what matters most for resilience: genetics, early (including prenatal) experiences, intelligence, schooling, the encouragement and social support a person receives, or their lifetime education.

Formal education is not the only path to cognitive reserve. A job which is challenging (but not overwhelming); leisure activities such as gardening, singing, or playing an instrument; volunteering; learning a language or reading a newspaper—all may help if done long-term, especially if done in company. Socializing is far more stimulating than people tend to realize. Lack of socializing, when it is felt as loneliness, is a big risk factor for dementia, as it is for other mental and physical illnesses (an effect observed both in high-income and developing countries). Good long-term relationships with family, partners, and friends also seem to buffer the risk of cognitive decline.

As with many other risk factors for dementia, these are modifiable—to an extent. Individuals can do a certain amount to help themselves maintain their brain resilience, but factors beyond their control, such as bereavement, can make it hard to keep up healthy habits, including social contact. That is especially the case when a person is hampered by one of the most challenging conditions we humans have to deal with: mental ill-health, and in particular, depression.

Depression

Depression is about more than feeling down. It involves cognitive changes too, including poorer memory and slowed thinking. It also features bodily changes. As with other so-called mental illnesses, effects are not restricted to the brain.

One of the hottest topics in current depression research is the link with inflammation. We all know how bad we can feel when fighting off an infection: low mood, lethargic, withdrawn, uninterested. Depression takes those feelings to extremes: despair, severe fatigue, alienation, and social isolation, every pleasure sucked out of existence. Could sickness and depression share physiological mechanisms? The hypothesis gained support when clinicians treating cancer began trialling a pro-inflammatory cytokine, interferon-alpha. The side-effects of this early immunotherapy included catastrophic depression.

More recently, research has found that many people with depression show signs of chronically elevated cytokines, and that those with such inflammatory markers tend to be less responsive to traditional anti-depressants. A meta-analysis of studies looking at anti-cytokine treatments found significant evidence that they also had anti-depressant effects. This has opened up new opportunities for treating depression.

Epidemiological studies have linked long-term depression, and other mental disorders such as schizophrenia, to a raised risk of developing dementia. However, reverse causation may yet again apply, at least when the depression happens later in life. Mood disturbances often accompany dementia from long before the condition is diagnosed. That does not necessarily rule out early-life depression being a risk factor (as some research has suggested). It may be that some varieties of depression, such as those involving inflammation, contribute more to dementia risk than others.

Again and again we see how risk factors interweave. Socializing, keeping mentally and physically active, good self-care, and having strong close relationships are protective against depression. Illness and loneliness can cause it, or be caused by it, not least because they make socializing and keeping active more difficult. The same web of influences also affects dementia risk.

Themes and variations

One way to think of this complexity is as involving a number of biological processes which can be varied by genetic, environmental, or other physiological risk factors. For example, if someone cuts their finger, their immune system triggers a well-coordinated suite of healing mechanisms to repair the wound—and that healing process is similar in humans across the world. Genetic differences may affect how fast a person heals; age and general health will also play a part; and so will how the injury is treated. But these are variations on a single, evolutionarily ancient theme: the biology of wound-healing.

The interweaving of genetic, environmental, and physiological risk factors that leads to dementia is a much harder scientific challenge. Not only are the variations much more numerous and intricate, but we aren't yet sure of all the themes and how they interact. Inflammation, vascular and heart function, blood sugar regulation, and oxidative stress are undoubtedly biological processes that, presumably, are similar worldwide. But as well as influencing each other, they all affect and are affected by genes, what else is going on in the body, and the physical, mental, and social environment—and those can vary considerably between people.

This may sound demoralizing, but it is actually good news for dementia research. To find out what causes any phenomenon, scientists need it—and its supposed causes—to vary, so that they can work out which changes go together. And the science of dementia has a huge, and still largely untapped, reservoir of variation, in that most of the research to date has been done in high-income, mainly Western countries. This is now changing, and as I mentioned at the start of this chapter, even initial basic assessments of prevalence and incidence are discovering a variety of patterns. They presumably reflect much greater variation in risk factors than is found in the restricted arena of Western science. The wider range offers researchers the hope of better understanding how risk factors affect neurodegeneration.

For example, Caucasian individuals who have the *APOE4* variant are more likely to get dementia, and get it earlier, than those who aren't carriers. In sub-Saharan Africans such as the Nigerian Yoruba this doesn't seem to be the case; but *APOE4* does seem to be a risk factor for African Americans. In India, dementia prevalence is below the global average; yet South Asians are more likely to have certain risk factors for dementia, such as diabetes, stroke, and heart disease. Dementia rates are rising in Latin America but seem to be falling in some Western countries. Stroke rates are rising in China, while falling in the West. In Japan, dementia rates have risen sharply since the country's diet became much more Westernized; and cross-cultural research has linked variation in the amount of meat eaten with variation in rates of Alzheimer's. High blood pressure and obesity are becoming more common in developing countries.

Other factors are also relevant. Environmental pollutants and smoking vary greatly between nations; so do social attitudes to dementia. Countries have started recognizing the illness as a social priority at different times, depending on their economic and cultural priorities, demographic changes, and so on. They differ in how well they identify people with dementia, and in how effectively they manage its medical risk factors, like high blood pressure or diabetes. Treatment for dementia itself also differs. The USA relies heavily on biomedicine and institutionalization. In China, on the other hand, most care still happens in the home, and many people with dementia use traditional Chinese medicines, not Western drugs. In China and India, perhaps a tenth of people with dementia lack social support; in Latin America, the figure may be up to a quarter.

Many small causes?

One downside of having so many interacting factors is that we cannot pull out one 'Factor X' and say, 'Here! X causes dementia, so all you have to do is alter X.' Another, as anyone who has experienced it will know, is that good health is hard to regain, once lost. Chronic illnesses make other illnesses more likely, pushing people into a quagmire they can't escape, however hard they work at lifestyle changes. Conversely, the upside for healthier folk is that making even one small lifestyle change may trigger a virtuous spiral, making the next steps easier to take.

In a human neighbourhood, many small things come together to make it a nice or nasty, safe or dangerous, enjoyable or stressful place to live. Areas that feel good have flourishing transport and communications links, a healthy and secure environment, reliable energy and food supplies, and plenty of activities. These affect residents differently depending on their background, their genes, their mental and physical health, and what else is going on in their lives.

Likewise, in a human brain, many things contribute to raising or lowering an individual brain cell's vulnerability to ageing. Most cases of dementia will have lots of small causes, jointly contributing towards the exact features, spread, and timing of the condition. This is why every case is unique to the person it affects.

Since the original amyloid cascade hypothesis was proposed, a wealth of research has uncovered many possible causes for dementia. What we still do not know is how much each cause contributes to the outcome; that is, which of them, alone or in combination, can push a brain from healthy ageing into disease. Must something, or several somethings, malfunction? Or can the characteristic changes of growing old—immune failings, oxidative stress, vascular problems, and so on—be enough to send a brain spiralling into neurodegeneration? To put it another way, we do not know whether every human being would get dementia if only they lived long enough, or whether only some have the particular factors which create the condition.

Many people, after all, do not live long enough, despite our increasing lifespans. They die of something else, like heart disease or infection: some other organ or body system collapsing before the brain does.

Changing the system

In theory, the study of risk factors in dementia points to a clear two-pronged strategy. First, detect and treat people with relevant health issues—like depression, high blood pressure, or diabetes—as early as possible. Second, try to stop people falling into ill-health in the first place. In practice, any such approach is beset by limited resources and by a wider failure of governments and other agencies to tackle causes rather than treat symptoms. Telling someone in poverty that they should eat a better diet, someone living with noisy neighbours that they should sleep better, or someone who drinks to blot out terrible memories that they should stop—because otherwise they might, decades later, get dementia—is unlikely to succeed. Yet this 'educational' approach is a healthcare system default. It looks and feels like doing something constructive, while respecting individual freedom. And it is a great deal cheaper than addressing the underlying problems of poverty, antisocial behaviour, and abuse. Health education does have benefits. It's just that—in another demonstration of the Matthew effect—they flow primarily to those who need them least.

Traditional thinking about healthcare exacerbates the problem. In future centuries—perhaps even future decades—people will look back dismayed at the crudity of current treatments for major illnesses. One-size-fits-all medications, often with nasty side-effects, sometimes given out without so much as a face-to-face meeting or blood test, let alone any attempt to personalize the treatment to the individual. They are the heritage of a view of healthcare as emergency response, not lifelong management.

Many healthcare systems are now adept at treating acute emergencies: broken bones, heart attacks, infections, fast-growing cancers. However, such treatments are not cost-free, either economically or physically. They can affect future health, sometimes profoundly, as many chemotherapy patients and heart attack survivors discover. As rates of heart disease, infections, and some cancers drop, attention is turning to the question of how to help survivors survive better, avoiding ruined health and the poor quality of life which accompanies it. The shift is under way towards a system geared to helping patients with multiple long-term diseases to live well, and perhaps regain some measure of health. It is sorely needed, and will greatly benefit people with dementia.

For the population overall, for most of whom dementia is a future possibility rather than a lived experience, the more behavioural changes they can make the better. Relying solely on individual will-power is not, however, likely to be effective. Indeed, it can be counterproductive: a distraction dangled by vested interests who don't want to change their ways, delaying structural changes while making people feel bad. Raised public awareness of the dangers of smoking was backed with taxation, plain packaging, government campaigns, and a ban on smoking in public places, together with the offer of alternatives such as nicotine replacement therapies and vaping. And still many people smoke.

Behavioural changes by the individual need supportive action from other agencies, such as the food industry (who are already taking some actions to, for example, cut salt and sugar, but who resist other tactics such as clearer 'traffic-light' labelling). With concerted societal effort, we could improve our diet, activity levels, and education, while reducing stress levels and exposure to pollution.

There is also evidence that people who see ageing in more positive terms tend to experience better ageing. If so, raising public awareness of the benefits of getting older—and the idea that dementia is something to live with, not die from—is worthwhile for everyone, not just people with dementia. Advertising and the media can play a major role here, since we learn much more from them than they explicitly tell us (like how the powers that be think about older people). Even small changes in how dementia and ageing are portrayed can have a big impact.

But what if you, or people close to you, are already showing symptoms of cognitive decline? In Chapter 5, we turn to diagnosis and treatment.

Chapter 5
Diagnosis and treatment

I mislaid my bank cards the other day. Not for the first time.
You've probably had similar experiences; perhaps you made a
joke of them. Many people do. But if someone is becoming
seriously worried about memory lapses, or getting lost in familiar
places—or if a person they know is acting out of character, or
showing signs of disorganized thought and speech—then they may
decide it's time to look for help.

My memory's dreadful. What next?

Like cancer before it, dementia used to be something people didn't
talk about. Not now. Charities work to raise awareness. News
features discuss statistics, potential drugs, or how to fund social
care for the elderly. Politicians launch challenges and national
strategies: to find a cure, improve diagnosis, coordinate better
treatment. Websites provide guides to help people facing the
challenge of living with or caring for someone with dementia.
(A list of useful websites is given at the end of this book.) And the
voices of those at the heart of all this activity are increasingly
being heard, reminding the rest of us that dementia is an illness to
be lived with, and one that can be lived with well. (For compelling
examples, including marathon runners, see the blog posts on
the 'Dementia Revolution' website, <https://www.
alzheimersresearchuk.org/dementia-revolution/>.)

For most people, the first step is to face the fear and think about whether they want to seek a formal diagnosis. There are advantages to doing this sooner rather than later. Anxiety is a major stressor, and knowing—even knowing the worst—can come as a relief (it is rarely a surprise). It can also bring families and friends together as they work out how to adapt. Clinicians can offer advice and support, as well as encouraging lifestyle alterations which may help to slow disease progression. Joining a research trial or support group might be beneficial. And if a diagnosis comes early enough, there may be medications available to ease symptoms and slow the decline. Then there will be more time to plan for the future. Adaptations to the home, financial and care planning, advance directives, power of attorney, and so on allow a person with dementia to exert more control over their illness and its impact on them.

In short, an early diagnosis gives the person more freedom to make choices, both about their life's ending and how to live beforehand. Delaying can raise difficult issues, for example around consent. (Can someone be said to have agreed to, say, moving into a care home if one minute later they've no recollection of ever having done so?) That said, some people are never formally diagnosed, or never learn their diagnosis. This is the path my family chose when our elderly relative, hospitalized after a fall, was given her label of vascular dementia. As far as I know, she was never told she had dementia, though I suspect she guessed the truth at times.

Symptom masking

My relative's deep familiarity with her house, her long-established patterns of life in a small village, and the fact that family members were handling shopping, finances, and suchlike, allowed her to hide her symptoms—perhaps even from herself. From the family too; human beings are good at not seeing what we don't want to have to face. Strangers engaged in casual chat might easily have judged her to be just a very old lady, frail of course, but managing. Only a longer conversation would have revealed the repetition, the stereotyped responses, the lost look I sometimes saw in her eyes.

Relying on routine and familiarity to mask dysfunction can complicate diagnosis. As US medics James E. Galvin and Carl H. Sadowsky wrote in 2012, 'physicians need to be wary of patients' ability to hide their symptoms. In the early stages of dementia, accommodation to or denial of changes in cognition, functional ability, mood, or behavior are common coping strategies. As the person's denial strengthens, the concerns of the family become more pressing, with the physician often caught in between and faced with apparently irreconcilable needs.'

No serious chronic illness is something an individual just has, or is afflicted by. It is something they live with, which changes them as they adapt to its daily fluctuations and more gradual developments. That adaptation takes time—years, often. It is experienced by both the person with dementia and those around them.

The path to diagnosis

Once the decision has been made to ask the question, the first step is towards primary healthcare: a local doctor. Their job is to make sure there is no obvious—and treatable—reason for the problems, such as thyroid dysfunction, B-vitamin deficiency, infection, or depression. Sometimes they may arrange additional tests, like an MRI or CT scan to rule out brain tumours and suchlike. If they find nothing, they should then decide which specialist the person should see next, and whether that referral should happen immediately. Depending on the patient's age and circumstances, the specialist is likely to be either someone trained to work with the elderly (a psychiatrist or geriatrician) or a neurologist.

If someone takes a cognitive test and passes easily, but is still seriously concerned, it is worth them saying so. The tests are a low bar, especially for people who are well educated or have had a high-powered job. (A 2018 study ran three commonly used tests on people whose dementia status was already known, and found that in a third of cases, one or more of the assessments got the status wrong.) If in doubt, ask for a referral. The reverse also applies; a person can appeal a diagnosis. A few years ago, another of my relatives was told by her GP that she had dementia, only to have the next level up—a consultant neurologist—inform her that it was in fact ataxia. (At the time, I recall, we felt reprieved. We have since learned that each kind of neurodegeneration has its own particular pattern of cruelties.)

Defining illness

A diagnosis of dementia can look like a threshold: a person has it or they don't. (Losing your keys now and again does not get you anywhere near the threshold, since it is not a major functional impairment, though in the morning rush it may momentarily feel like it. Persistently getting lost when you go shopping is another matter.) Yet as ever with this condition, things aren't so simple. To see why, we need to look at how dementia is classified.

Two major systems are used to classify brain disorders. One, from the WHO, also deals with other diseases; it is the *ICD* (*International Classification of Diseases*). The other, from the USA, is the *DSM* (*Diagnostic and Statistical Manual*), which focuses on psychiatric and neurological conditions. Both have been around for decades—the *ICD* for over a century—and in recent years their authors have collaborated to make them more similar. Both have been revised periodically to reflect society's changing ideas of what counts as illness. (Homosexuality, for example, was removed from the *DSM* in 1973 and replaced by the unloved compromise 'sexual orientation disturbance'. In 1987, this too was ditched.)

For dementia, the major change has been from seeing it in terms of a simple threshold to seeing it as a spectrum of gradually worsening symptoms. In the current *DSM-5*, for example, severe dementia and memory loss, and mild cognitive impairment (MCI), are now called major, and mild, 'neurocognitive disorder'. This acknowledges the grey areas of cognitive impairment, and the difficulty of diagnosing early-stage dementia. It also emphasizes the role of social cognitive deficits. And it highlights the importance of functional impairment severe enough to significantly hamper daily living. Often the line between mild and major NCD—MCI and dementia—is a matter of fine clinical judgement: not just 'How much is this person struggling?' but 'How much support do they have?' and 'How do they feel about the treatments I can offer?' The idea of a spectrum of cognitive dysfunction makes sense of what clinicians have long known.

But it does more. As James E. Galvin wrote in 2017, 'dementia may be a disorder that develops over a lifetime'. In other words, the spectrum model extends the time range, accommodating the idea of pre-clinical disease. That idea is controversial. The debate is not over whether the brain changes exist, but whether a bodily state should be considered 'illness' if the people who have it can still manage their lives well and may not even have noticed any symptoms. Hence the importance of biomarkers.

When diagnosing, clinicians try to distinguish whether the cognitively impaired person has some form of dementia, or whether their symptoms result from some other neurological, or bodily, cause which might require different treatment. As we have seen, an infection elsewhere, such as in the urinary tract, can affect the brain's function, causing confusion or delirium that can resemble dementia. Late-life depression, or neurodegenerative disorders like ataxia, can also look similar (as with my relative whose ataxia was interpreted as dementia). All three can involve apathy, agitation and emotional volatility, apparent personality change, problems with everyday tasks, reduced mobility, and so on.

Diagnosis and treatment

109

Timing also matters. Generally, dementia symptoms are insidious, differentiating them from sudden-onset impairment caused by, say, delirium or encephalitis; but there are exceptions. Vascular dementia, for example, can sometimes become apparent after a stroke.

Domains of dementia

Dementia's typically gradual onset is part of what makes it so hard to diagnose early; and as noted earlier, distinguishing between types of dementia is a further challenge—even post-mortem, let alone in the clinic. Getting an accurate diagnosis of, say, Lewy body dementia or Alzheimer's is important, however, because medications used to treat dementia symptoms may have differing effects on different types. How, and how fast, dementia progresses also varies by type, so a specific diagnosis can help people understand what to expect. Up to a point: individuals vary greatly in how their illness unfolds.

To explore the differences between varieties of dementia, let us look at what one of the standard references, *DSM-5*, says about 'major neurocognitive disorder' (NCD). It identifies and discusses thirteen subtypes, distinguishing them by their patterns of deficits across six groups of mental functions, known as 'neurocognitive domains'. These are:

- Complex attention. More than just noticing things, this includes the ability to stay focused and multitask. NCDs affecting this domain can manifest as distractibility, slower thinking, and being quickly overwhelmed by complex tasks like mentally adding up figures.

- Executive function. Often thought of as planning and decision-making, this also includes mental flexibility and self-control. NCDs can impair a person's ability to override habitual or instinctive responses, and reduce the ability to learn from feedback.

- Learning and memory. As Alzheimer's notes on Auguste Deter showed, recent memory can be profoundly affected by NCDs. Symptoms include repetitive conversations, rapidly forgetting new information, and the inability to remember one's intentions for long enough to carry them out.

- Language. Both understanding and using language can be affected, sometimes so severely that in late-stage dementia the person may no longer speak at all. Typical NCD symptoms in earlier stages include problems with finding words, putting sentences together, or naming things.

- Perceptual-motor. Deficits in this domain often affect the ability to use familiar objects, navigate familiar routes, and make sense of a space when it looks different (e.g. towards sundown). Hallucinations, and problems controlling movements, may also feature.

- Social cognition. This domain includes theory of mind, empathy, morality, and emotion recognition and control. NCDs affecting it can lead to disorders of mood and motivation, or to social deficits ranging from awkwardness to frankly antisocial behaviour. The *DSM* notes that people affected often have little or no insight into their condition.

To be diagnosed with a major NCD, the equivalent of dementia, people must be so seriously impaired in one or more domains that their performance on cognitive testing is at least two standard deviations below the average; that is, in the lowest 2.5 per cent of the population. (For mild NCDs the criterion is between one and two standard deviations below average, covering the next 13.5 per cent of the population.) To rule out developmental disabilities, a person's performance must have become significantly worse than it used to be, as judged by them, by a clinician, or by a 'knowledgeable informant' like a spouse or partner. The problems must be severe enough to 'interfere with independence in everyday activities' (*DSM-5*, p. 602). And the dysfunction must not be due either to delirium, or to some other disorder such as major depression.

Performance on the six domains is key to a *DSM-5* diagnosis of dementia, but there are other criteria too. For example, there may be a known genetic mutation present (e.g. in young-onset Alzheimer's or frontotemporal dementia) or evidence of brain changes from neuroimaging (e.g. in Alzheimer's, frontotemporal, or vascular dementia). These can help clinicians to decide which subtype is the most appropriate, though many people will have features of more than one. Depending on how many criteria are met, the clinician may diagnose 'probable' or 'possible' major (or mild) NCD.

The usual suspects

In *DSM-5*, the five most common and familiar varieties of dementia are named Alzheimer's disease, frontotemporal lobar degeneration, Lewy body disease, vascular disease, and a subtype 'due to multiple etiologies' (i.e. more than one cause; elsewhere it's known as 'mixed dementia'). Together these make up around 95 per cent of dementia cases. (The *DSM* does not currently include the recently described 'LATE' type, mentioned in Chapter 3 and thought to be caused by the TDP-43 protein.)

For Alzheimer's, clinicians describe the onset of the illness as insidious and its progress as gradual. It's often impossible to pin down when symptoms began, and the neurocognitive problems get worse slowly (unlike, say, stroke or delirium). The affected domains must include learning and memory. Executive function is often impaired, but social cognition may be relatively spared long into the course of the illness. If the condition worsens steadily, and there's no evidence of other causes (e.g. stroke), then other possibilities like vascular dementia can be provisionally ruled out.

Frontotemporal lobar degeneration, commonly known as frontotemporal dementia (FTD), is also insidious in onset and gradual in progression; but unlike Alzheimer's, it tends to spare learning and memory. It also tends to worsen more rapidly, and affect younger people, compared with Alzheimer's or vascular dementia. In some cases of FTD, language is the neurocognitive domain most affected. In others, as we saw in Chapter 1, the disease mainly targets social cognition and executive function; it can also alter eating habits. In this 'behavioural variant' form, visual function tends to be less impaired, but parkinsonian symptoms are notable. Indeed, as well as being a diagnosis in its own right, FTD can accompany other neurodegenerative disorders with severe movement problems, such as motor neuron disease, progressive supranuclear palsy, and corticobasal degeneration.

Lewy body disease is a term that covers several neurodegenerative conditions; I will focus here on DLB. In this form of dementia, as in Alzheimer's, vascular, and FTD, symptoms tend to affect executive function and attention. Learning and memory, and social cognition, are less affected. Perceptual-motor problems, on the other hand, are prominent: as I noted in Chapter 1, DLB is characterized by hallucinations and parkinsonian symptoms. Falls, blackouts, and sleep disorders are frequent. Also distinctive is that cognitive function fluctuates considerably over time. Clinicians cannot rely on a single assessment session to rule this type of dementia in or out, so 'knowledgeable informants' are crucial.

Diagnosing DLB correctly is especially important because this type of dementia is often accompanied by a highly dangerous symptom: sensitivity to neuroleptic drugs (antipsychotics). Though generally not recommended, these powerful chemicals are widely used to treat symptoms of dementia; but they can lead to adverse reactions including tremor, rigidity, agitation, excessive sedation, fever, and confusion. In DLB, severe neuroleptic sensitivity may affect up to half of people who have it—and the reactions can be fatal. Hence the need for accurate diagnosis.

Vascular dementia can be hard to distinguish from Alzheimer's, especially early on and if neuroimaging is not available. Both subtypes tend to affect memory while the NCD is still at the mild stage, with executive function, attention, language, and perceptual-motor deficits becoming more prominent as the disease progresses, and social cognitive function being relatively well preserved. Unlike Alzheimer's, however, vascular dementia tends to progress unevenly: a sudden worsening of symptoms (due to new strokes or mini-strokes) may be followed by a long period of little change. DLB can have similar 'plateaus' in cognition, but levels of alertness in vascular dementia do not fluctuate as much as in DLB. The way problems develop in vascular and frontotemporal dementia can also look similar in some domains (e.g. executive function) but the behavioural problems so common in FTD are not typical of vascular disease, though emotional volatility can be. To diagnose the condition, there must be sufficient evidence of cerebrovascular disease (CVD), such as a medical history of strokes or transient ischaemic attacks. Neuroimaging (if available) can confirm that CVD is present, and—as with stroke—there are often signs of physical disability.

Rarer subtypes

Although genetic and neuroimaging evidence is available for some of the more common dementia subtypes, they are defined in *DSM-5* by their clinical symptoms. Among the *DSM*'s thirteen categories of NCD, however, are six rarer subtypes, all of which are identified by their presumed cause. (At the start of the NCDs chapter, its authors note that causal links are firmer for NCDs than for any other kind of condition in the *DSM*, thanks to the vast research literature.) I have already mentioned three of these aetiologies: traumatic brain injury (in Chapter 4), prion disease (in Chapter 2), and substance/medicinal use (the example of alcohol in Chapter 1). *DSM-5* also lists NCDs associated with Parkinson's disease, Huntington's disease, and HIV infection.

Among people with Parkinson's, 'as many as 75% will develop a major NCD sometime in the course of their disease' (*DSM-5*, p. 637).

As with vascular dementia, mood disorders often feature. However, so do hallucinations and sleep disorders, making this form of dementia look very like DLB. Both are classed as 'Lewy body disease'; but in DLB, parkinsonian symptoms appear after the onset of dementia, whereas in Parkinsonian dementia the Parkinson's begins before the dementia (by convention, at least a year before).

Similarly, in Huntington's dementia, either Huntington's disease or a known genetic risk for it must be present before the onset of dementia.

Both Parkinson's and Huntington's dementia, like Alzheimer's, are insidious in onset and gradual in progression. They commonly feature anxiety, depression, and apathy as well as problems with attention, executive function, and memory. Huntington's dementia may also lead people to develop obsessions.

In 'NCD associated with HIV infection', the virus can get into the brain, reproduce inside microglia, and cause them to pump out cytokines, damaging and eventually killing neurons. Memory and language tend to be less affected, executive function and speed of processing more so. Modern treatments for HIV infection have greatly reduced its impact, and fewer than 5 per cent of people with HIV now reach the threshold for a major NCD. This form of dementia is unusual in its patterns over time. Symptoms may worsen gradually, but they may also be stable, or fluctuate (without worsening with time, unlike DLB), or even improve. Diagnosis requires not only known HIV infection, but also ruling out other infections and brain cancer. These can result from HIV's suppression of the immune system, but they are not due to HIV directly affecting the brain.

Finally, for those rare cases that do not fit with any of the above, *DSM-5* concludes with two catch-all subtypes: NCD associated with another medical condition, and unspecified NCD.

After diagnosis

If someone does get a formal diagnosis of dementia, they should expect to be told the type of dementia they have, its typical course and impact, and how to access support—especially if they are living alone with the illness. They should get advice, verbal and written, about steps to take to make life easier, about driving if they're a motorist, and about advance planning. Help for carers, and information about rights, should also be clearly signposted. (For more information, see the list of useful organizations.) After diagnosis, the person is likely to be sent back to their primary care physician, who should regularly check up on them thereafter.

Being diagnosed with any form of dementia can be immensely stressful. Quite apart from the challenges they bring, these are widely feared and stigmatized conditions. Yet to put dementia in a separate category is to downplay its similarities to other serious illnesses. They too change the people who endure them, sometimes profoundly. Coming face to face with death and frailty can force someone to grow up, for example, or reassess what really matters. A diagnosis of dementia is usually not The End, but the start of something that will not always or only be difficult. There is still living to be done, enjoyment to be had, autonomy to be exercised.

In most cases of dementia, what goes first is what matters less for identity: recent memories, money management, the ability to plan. The emotions, more basic to who we are, last longer: a person with dementia can still feel frightened—or loved—long into the illness. It is a gradual withdrawal from life, letting go of the least important things first. With luck, and good care, the farewell can be (mostly) gentle.

Good care is person-centred, not one-size-fits-all. It focuses on what the individual can do instead of commenting on what they can't do. It remembers that even the most immobile face hides a mind still able to feel pain, anxiety, and humiliation. And it respects the humanity and dignity of the person, however ill, rather than reducing them to their medical condition. Unfortunately, good care requires resources of time, energy, and funding that are not always available. A 2016 review of medical outcomes for nearly two million patients—with and without dementia, mostly in the USA—found that those with the condition fared worse: higher rates of readmission, complications, dehydration, heart problems, and death, coupled with less use of medical procedures such as ventilation and intensive care.

A study from Ireland, also published in 2016, pointed to possible reasons. It looked at how hospitals assessed elderly patients and found that both their cognitive assessments and staff dementia training were 'sub-optimal'. In the same year, the UK's Royal College of Psychiatrists was collecting data for an audit of hospital care for people with dementia. Its report, published in 2017, found that, while care was beginning to improve, there was a long way to go, especially around issues of consent and communication, detecting delirium, and providing good nutrition.

At present, neither care nor any other treatment can reverse neurodegeneration. There are ways, however, to make the process more tolerable, and perhaps even slow down cognitive decline. Both pharmaceutical and behavioural options are available. I'll begin with drugs—current and potential—and then look at other approaches.

Standard drugs

As we have seen, lifestyle changes to improve general health may be beneficial. At the least, ensuring adequate food and drink, stable routines, and good company can have a surprisingly positive effect, especially on elderly people who live alone. If a diagnosis of Alzheimer's comes early enough, however, there are also pharmacological options: the four standard treatments currently available. As we have seen, donepezil, galantamine, and rivastigmine work by suppressing the enzyme which breaks down the neurotransmitter acetylcholine. Memantine affects glutamate signalling. Which if any is prescribed will depend on the person's symptoms, how they feel about taking drugs, and how well they can tolerate the side-effects.

Other medications may be prescribed for specific symptoms, such as agitation or sleep problems, as well as for other illnesses. For example, anti-psychotics such as risperidone are sometimes used for severe behavioural problems, like aggression, or psychological symptoms, like hallucinations. These drugs however can have heavy-duty side-effects (as we saw with neuroleptic sensitivity in DLB), so should be used only temporarily and as a last resort.

Prescribing in older people has to be done carefully. Not only do they tend to have more medical conditions—and hence more medicines, which may interact in unpredicted ways—but ageing bodies and brains may respond differently to drugs compared with younger ones. Of course, all drugs on the market have been safety-tested in clinical trials on volunteers, but unless the drug is specifically targeting a disease of old age, those volunteers may well have been young, healthy adults, not senior citizens. We do not yet know enough about how ageing affects bodily reactions to drugs prescribed for other problems, especially when those drugs are combined, and when they themselves affect cognition, as some medications do.

That said, technological advances now enable researchers to mass-screen candidate chemicals for interference with biological pathways. The hope is that as drug development gets more efficient, new drugs will be more specific and less likely to cause severe side-effects.

Potential drugs

In late 2018, I did a search of the US ClinicalTrials.gov website for 'Alzheimer Disease'. It found 1,958 trials, of which 591 were ongoing. Of these latter, some are descriptive—testing new neuroimaging tracers and suchlike. Just over three-quarters (454) list at least one specific intervention. Half of the intervention trials are testing either drugs (213 trials), or biological compounds such as antibodies, stem cells, or biomarkers (18 trials). Almost a fifth (19.8 per cent) are testing behavioural approaches, such as music or laughter therapy. Dietary supplements are listed as the intervention in 3.3 per cent. The remaining quarter are using other methods—from questionnaires and PET scans, to 'smart' insoles and activity monitors, to radiation and even gene therapy—to assess and treat their volunteers. (How interventions are categorized overlaps, so for example a trial listed as 'drug' may include antibody treatment, or may compare a drug with a behavioural therapy.)

Of the 213 intervention studies categorized as drug trials, some are testing traditional Alzheimer's therapies such as memantine or donezepil. Others target the amyloid or tau proteins, either by using some form of immunotherapy (e.g. antibodies, vaccines), or by interfering with their processing (e.g. inhibiting synthesis or aggregation), or by altering their effects (e.g. disrupting the action of amyloid oligomers).

Beyond these well-known approaches, the ClinicalTrials.gov database reveals a fine array of other potential ways to treat dementia, some deriving from clinical observations, others from basic research into particular brain mechanisms. For example, some drugs have been chosen to treat specific symptoms, such as agitation. How such treatments work is not well understood, but they can help treat agitation in other patients, so the trial aims to learn whether they also help people with dementia.

Sometimes the drug was originally designed to treat an illness other than dementia—such as epilepsy (e.g. gabapentin) or diabetes (insulin)—but is now being repurposed for neurodegeneration.

One trial is giving infusions of blood plasma proteins. (Those 'vampire senior' headlines may yet return.) The physiological effects of young blood on aged mice are not well understood, but they seem beneficial, so the next step is to see what transfusions do to elderly humans.

Then there are pharmaceuticals targeting specific pathways. The database includes drugs affecting neurotransmitters and hormones—such as glutamate, noradrenaline, and angiotensin—as well as drugs targeting mitochondrial and other intracellular functions.

Of course, even where a drug's main action is known, it may have other effects as well. The database also lists trials involving statins, anti-psychotics, and antidepressants, as well as dietary extracts (grapeseed, ginkgo, essential fatty acids). Some effects of these chemicals are known, but their effects on neurodegeneration, if any, are not clear. Hence the trials.

Non-drug treatments

Unless they join a clinical trial (and are assigned to the treatment rather than the placebo group), people with cognitive problems are probably years away from accessing most of the drugs being currently tested. Where a person lives, their economic status, their government's attitudes to healthcare spending, even their doctor's beliefs about dementia—as well as their own—will affect how early they are diagnosed and which if any drugs are then prescribed. However, even if pharmaceuticals are not available there are other ways to improve people's quality of life, as we have seen. These include 'non-pharmacological interventions' (NPIs), some of which have been tested in residential settings and at home. Some of these have been found to be as helpful as, or even more helpful than, drugs.

Found, how? The gold standard for drug testing is the double-blind randomized controlled trial (RCT), in which volunteers are randomly assigned to receive either the candidate drug or a placebo. (Some trials also include a group getting treatment-as-usual.) The idea is that if the treatment and control groups are big enough, they will not differ in any significant respect, such as average age, educational background, or gender balance. Importantly, both the volunteers and the people running the trial do not know (are blind to) who is getting treatment and who placebo. Only at the end of the trial will the scientists break the codes and analyse the data. In a good trial, they will also set out how they plan to analyse the data, and what counts as success, before the trial begins, and register the trial so that others know to expect results in due course. (Clinical trials which do not report their findings, often because the outcomes were not as expected, are a huge waste of money and can be a medical hazard. Estimates suggest that about half of trials do not publish their data.)

RCTs work well for drugs, where a placebo pill or injection can be indistinguishable from treatment to the person who receives it—although side-effects can sometimes break the blinding. It is not so easy to provide a good placebo for NPIs, not least because it is usually obvious who has been assigned to, say, music therapy and who has not. Furthermore, NPIs change more than one variable. Instead of adding a single chemical to a person's intake, an NPI alters their routine, how much attention and social interaction they get, how much moving and talking they do, and so on. Which is the effective change, or is it all of them? Comparing multiple NPIs, such as music and art therapy, is often done, but it doesn't altogether resolve the problems.

With these points noted, and bearing in mind the familiar scientific cry of 'More research needed', what do we know about

NPIs so far? Recent years have seen increasing numbers of trials for behavioural treatments: when I looked, the ClinicalTrials.gov database listed ninety. They focus on education and cognitive skills, social and emotional support, exercise, diet and lifestyle changes, technologies, or specific interventions such as acupressure or speech therapy.

How NPIs are delivered varies. Some are bundled into overall or 'multicomponent' care programmes, which have been developed through experience of managing care homes. However, given that most people with dementia live in the community, not in residential care, some interventions address this, even to the extent of being provided online.

Then there is the question of who gets the intervention: the person with dementia (alone, or as part of a group), formal carers, or informal caregivers. Most NPI testing to date has been done in residential settings, but most care is provided informally, by at least one friend or family member. Some NPIs therefore address the needs of caregivers, or the care 'dyad' (for example, by changing interactions between the carer and the person cared for).

NPIs addressing education and cognitive skills range beyond simply providing educational support (information about dementia). Cognitive training, for example, aims to improve specific skills such as memory and attention, often using games. Cognitive stimulation therapy aims to get people thinking and doing activities based on a theme such as food, childhood, or word association. Unlike training, it is less focused on particular components of cognition, more holistic, and usually group-based.

According to a 2018 review of NPI research by Ann Kolanowski and colleagues, there is some evidence that educational support is helpful. For mild to moderate dementia, there is more evidence for cognitive stimulation therapy than for training. If training has benefits, these may be most apparent early on, for people with milder cognitive impairment. It is also not clear whether any improvement from training translates into practical enhancements of the ability to function in daily life.

Some approaches, accordingly, focus on cognitive rehabilitation, helping the person to deal with specific problems which arise when living with dementia. This highlights another issue in dementia care: it needs to be tailored both to the person and to the stage of cognitive impairment they have reached. Such tailoring can be difficult for close carers, not least because people adapt to situations and tend not to notice gradual changes. Sometimes symptoms can get worse abruptly: after a fall, or because of a stroke. But often the decline is so insidious that only formal processes, such as regular assessment, will reveal how much the dementia has progressed.

NPIs addressing social and emotional support include providing access to support groups or trained companions, training in emotion recognition and regulation, and forms of psychotherapy such as CBT (cognitive behavioural therapy), counselling, and occupational therapy. There is evidence that psychotherapy, added to usual care, can help people with dementia and their carers to manage the many non-cognitive symptoms of the condition and deal with its emotional challenges.

There is some evidence that physical exercise, especially when combined with other approaches and initiated early on, may be a helpful NPI. Likewise for dietary improvements, although the key word is 'dietary'; taking nutrient supplements does not appear to offer the same benefits. Sleep rhythms are often disturbed in dementia, which can make life very difficult for people—and their carers. Regular routines and good sleep hygiene may help to maintain more beneficial patterns.

Other lifestyle interventions also have evidence to support them, though the quality and amount varies greatly. Among the most rigorous assessments of such evidence are the frequent reviews published by the independent Cochrane organization, which summarize the state of the science on a topic. Cochrane reviews find some support for music therapy, reminiscence therapy, case management (which coordinates person-centred care), and functional analysis. (Functional analysis addresses challenging behaviours by asking why the person is reacting in such a way. Are they in pain, or feeling threatened? What unmet needs are driving the behaviour?)

There is much less evidence for personally tailored activities, light therapy for sleep problems, massage and touch, art therapy, assistive technologies for memory problems, sensory stimulation techniques such as pet therapy, and simulated presence therapy (i.e. playing recordings of close others to the person with dementia). A systematic review of Montessori-based methods for dementia found them helpful for problems with eating, but evidence for their effects on mood and cognition was unclear.

For caregivers, CBT has shown promise in relieving depression and stress. There is less evidence for mindfulness-based stress reduction, or for group or individually tailored interventions designed to help caregivers adjust to the transition from home to residential care. A 2018 meta-analysis by Jütten and colleagues of 'the effectiveness of psychosocial and behavioral interventions on burden, depression, anxiety, quality of life, stress, and sense of competence in informal dementia caregivers' concluded that there is evidence for impact on all of these measures, except for anxiety. However, such effects, though statistically significant, are small. The authors' summing up is stark. 'Clinical practice with informal caregivers should be aware of these findings: the interventions may aid the caregivers to some extent, but they may need more in order to be really helped in their caregiving role.'

The lack of good-quality evidence for many NPIs has to do with the quantity of available trials as well as the quality. As Kolanowski and colleagues point out, there is plenty of work to be done: not only on testing specific interventions, but on developing appropriate outcomes and tools for measuring them. Researchers are working to understand more about how NPIs affect brain function, and to make sure that improvements on outcome measures translate into better coping and quality of life. They need to take account of the type and stage of dementia, the situations in which people confront and adjust to their diagnosis, and the person's own likes and preferences. To quote from the Kolanowski article directly, 'The experience of the person living with dementia is virtually absent in the literature.'

Meanwhile, perhaps the content of the intervention may be less crucial than the way in which it is delivered. For example, a 2010 review in the journal *Psychogeriatrics*, by Haruyasu Yamaguchi and colleagues, offers five principles to guide NPIs (see Box 2).

Box 2 Five principles for non-pharmacological interventions

'(i) enjoyable and comfortable activities in an accepting atmosphere;

(ii) activities associated with empathetic two-way communication between the therapist and patient, as well as between patients;

(iii) therapists should praise patients to enhance motivation;

(iv) therapists should try to offer each patient some social role that takes advantage of his/her remaining abilities; and

(v) the activities should be based on errorless learning to ensure a pleasant atmosphere and to maintain a patient's dignity.'

In short, be gentle with, and value, yourself and those around you. It's a recipe for life, not just for dealing with dementia.

In Chapter 6, we'll look to the future.

Chapter 6
The future of dementia

Research

On the research front, the future for dementia looks exciting. Scientists have more tools than ever for understanding how neurodegeneration affects brains. Better neuroimaging techniques are being developed to detect key proteins like amyloid and tau, to image the brain in more detail, and to get a clearer picture of its connectivity. Bigger data sets are making conclusions more reliable. Advances in stem cell technologies and genetics offer the hope of personalized medicine, while work on epigenetics, RNA, and post-translation processing is revealing the complexity of nature–nurture interactions. Meanwhile, research on immunity and insulin, mitochondria and microglia, the blood–brain barrier, and more is revealing the extent to which neurodegeneration is affected by bodily as well as brain changes. The scientific challenges of dementia are exceptionally complex, but at least we now recognize that complexity.

Better still, dementia scientists now have the political wind in their sails, as the rich West starts to realize the economic and social impact of its ageing populations. And not just the West: Japan is a world leader on the issue. Funding for dementia research has long lagged behind resources for other major killers, but it is now at unprecedented levels.

Clinical trials based on the amyloid hypothesis have not yet delivered even treatments for Alzheimer's, let alone a cure. Nonetheless, many scientists are optimistic that disease-modifying treatments, based on this or other ideas about Alzheimer's, will be available before many more years have passed. It is unclear whether a cure for advanced neurodegeneration, which would require effectively regrowing large areas of brain tissue, could ever be possible. Yet even lesser treatments will be welcomed by the millions of people affected—provided they can afford them.

Care

While we wait for drugs to cure or treat dementia, one message from the science is very clear: prevention matters. Individuals and particularly societies can act to help themselves. Depending on our genes, history, and circumstances, looking after our brains may help us to avoid dementia altogether, or at least delay it. Moreover, we don't need to learn new rules-to-live-by, because the guidance is familiar: eat well, sleep well, exercise, keep busy, socialize, stay in touch with nature, and try to reduce exposure to stress, trauma, and dangerous substances in food, drink, and air. It is extremely difficult to achieve these aspirations to the degree of burnished perfection held up by some who promote them; but that need not deter us from attempting some improvement. It is much easier to make a small change, and then another, and another.

The hopeful mind-set of dementia science encourages us all not to give up. Where that mind-set can become a problem is if it sways us towards the hope of a quick fix, and a drug fix at that. Non-pharmaceutical interventions can be equally effective in helping people with dementia to live better lives. Whether those interventions are carried out by family, partners, nurses, or therapists, formally or informally, they rely on an assumption that the person with dementia, however advanced their condition, is still a person, deserving of the same respect and consideration of their dignity as any other human being.

In this sense, the old and terrifying idea that dementia strips its victims of their human essence—the self—is not the monolithic truth that makes people dread and stigmatize the condition. Rather, it is as true as we allow it to be. Much of the self is not lodged apart, in a single, aloof individual: no man is an island, women perhaps even less so. Most of what matters to people is found in the social bonds that make them known, accepted, and cared-for. Those bonds are bridges across the gaps between people that dementia opens up. The more we work on strengthening them, the longer they will serve us.

It follows that individuals cannot be held entirely responsible for their own health. Likewise, caring for those who are ill is best done as a social endeavour, not by leaving people to their own devices. (Currently, patients and families pay two-thirds of the costs of their illness, according to UK figures from the Alzheimer's Society.) Asking people with dementia what they want, as early as possible in the illness, is crucial to good person-centred care; and most people say that they would like to stay at home, as independent as they can be for as long as possible.

Unfortunately, and particularly in the West, this is not how the system has evolved. Current social care relies heavily on institutions, on a poorly paid workforce, and on the unpaid labour of informal carers. Institutions can be excellent—my family has been lucky in its choices—but years of underfunding have led many to close and left many more struggling. Homecare has also been pared back by austerity. As for the unpaid labour, the Alzheimer's Society values the work done by unpaid dementia carers in the UK at £11 billion annually. Alzheimer's Disease International estimates that, globally, 40 per cent of the total cost of dementia ($818 billion in 2015) goes on informal care. The costs are proportionately greater in low-income countries (69 per cent). High-income countries spend more on medical and social care; yet informal care still makes up 38 per cent of dementia care costs. (In the USA and Japan, the costs of informal care have been estimated at, respectively, around \$234 billion and 6 trillion yen.)

These are sizeable sums. The UK figure, for instance, is about a quarter of what the UK government spent on long-term sickness and disability benefits in 2018. Ironically, some government welfare spending is going to carers made ill themselves by the challenges of caring. This is more likely when the dementia includes behavioural and psychological symptoms such as agitation and aggression, or sleep disturbances. A highly stressed carer may involuntarily care less well, and that may in turn stress their patient and worsen symptoms. To stop the resulting vicious circle, it is essential that carers get adequate, and continuing, support from early on. It is also cheaper, in the long term. Unfortunately, many healthcare systems do not have the money to fund even the short-term 'stitch in time', let alone pay for dealing with the consequences when that stitch is left undone.

Care, and support for informal caregivers, is now widely recognized as a major problem, and one which is likely to increase as the global population ages. Prevention-based approaches may reduce the problem—in the long term. Between the here and now and that bright, brain-healthy future, however, is an unfortunate convergence of serious challenges with alarming implications. Not only are the demographics changing, but we are now starting to face up to the costs of the last two centuries' rush—especially in the West—to embrace life's modern conveniences.

Cheap food was a blessing, except that it may be damaging our health even early in life, both from the amounts we eat and the chemicals used in food production. Sewage systems saved uncounted lives, but the use of lead in the pipes (and in paint, petrol, and elsewhere) poisoned the water and impaired many people's cognition. Cars bestowed freedom and boosted economic growth, but their toxins have been polluting our brains for years. We have plastic particles in our bodies. And so on, up to and including climate change. We are poisoning ourselves, fighting over scarce resources, despoiling the oceans, driving other species to extinction, wrecking our soils, and exterminating the insects we need to pollinate our crops. It's adolescent, to say the least: behaving as if there are no consequences, no long term—as if only we in our present moment matter. And it's brain-damaging. As well as promoting neurodegeneration, it also impairs our intelligence, our capacity to reason—just when we need it most.

These global problems will get worse before they get better. So will the problems they have helped to cause, like rising numbers of people who need better dementia care. The question of how to fund the consequences of all those unwise choices—without entire healthcare systems buckling under the strain—is one of the most difficult of our age. Yet although there is a very tough period ahead, there is much that we as individuals—and citizens—can do to shorten the bad times and bring on a brighter future. We can look after our bodies, take part in clinical trials, and donate to research charities. We can volunteer, fundraise, or work to reduce stigma, and the stress on carers, in our own communities. We can cut down on driving and flying, campaign for cleaner air, demand that industries take better care of our food and the environment, lobby our governments to do more on climate change and conservation. The potential benefits extend well beyond a lower risk of dementia.

The more we understand about human brain health, the more we realize that even small changes, if there are enough of them, can tip a cell/brain/person towards catastrophe. Likewise, small moves to protect our brains can tip us away from neurodegeneration, especially if we form good habits early and stick to them. Many people are already taking steps, but we can all do more to reduce our risk of dementia—and our children's—and make life easier for those who already have it.

Will we take action? Reader, over to you.

References

Please note: the references listed here are only for major mentions in the text where further details are needed to track down the reference. More about research not specified here can be found in my 2016 book *The Fragile Brain* and in the 'Further reading' section. I have tried to use publicly available sources wherever possible, but unfortunately not all are yet open-access (as of March 2020). It may be worth checking the website, as more journals are yielding to the pressure to become open-access. Another good place to start is the searchable database of scientific literature PubMed (<https://pubmed.ncbi.nlm.nih.gov/>), which provides abstracts where available, and often the full text of a piece, as well as links to publisher websites.

Chapter 1: The challenges of dementia

The statistics on dementia prevalence are taken from Alzheimer's Disease International's World Alzheimer Report 2018, available from <https://www.alz.co.uk/research/world-report-2018>.

The WHO statistics on global disease prevalence, 2016, are taken from the Global Burden of Disease study (2016) cause-specific mortality estimates. Data are available from <http://www.who.int/healthinfo/global_burden_disease/estimates/en/>. A summary can be found at <http://www.who.int/gho/mortality_burden_disease/causes_death/top_10/en/>. The 2017 update was published in the *Lancet* in November 2018 (see e.g. D. Dicker et al. (2018), 'Global, regional, and national age-sex-specific mortality and life expectancy, 1950–2017: a systematic analysis for the Global Burden of Disease

Study 2017', *Lancet*, 392 (10159), 1684–735). The papers are available at <https://www.thelancet.com/gbd>. The analysis also provides a useful and fascinating set of data visualizations at <https://vizhub.healthdata.org/gbd-compare/>. For information comparing the top ten causes of death by national income level, see <https://www.who.int/news-room/fact-sheets/detail/the-top-10-causes-of-death>. As of 2016, dementia was third for high-income countries, fifth for upper-middle-income countries, and not in the top ten for lower-middle- or low-income countries.

Cicero, M. T. (1923), *De Senectute*. Cambridge, Mass., Loeb Classical Library: Harvard University Press. (Translations of *De Senectute* are available online, e.g. at <https://en.wikisource.org/wiki/Cicero_de_Senectute/Text>.)

The excerpts from Alzheimer's case notes in Chapters 1 and 2 are taken from K. Maurer, S. Volk, and H. Gerbaldo (1997), 'Auguste D and Alzheimer's disease', *Lancet*, 349 (9064), 1546–9. (This article is available free online with registration from <https://www.thelancet.com/journals/lancet/article/PIIS0140-6736(96)10203-8/fulltext>.)

Katzman, R. (1976), 'The prevalence and malignancy of Alzheimer disease: a major killer', *Archives of Neurology*, 33 (4), 217–18. (This editorial is available from <https://jamanetwork.com/journals/jamaneurology/article-abstract/574311>, but is not open-access.)

Selvackadunco, S., et al. (2019), 'Comparison of clinical and neuropathological diagnoses of neurodegenerative diseases in two centres from the Brains for Dementia Research (BDR) cohort', *Journal of Neural Transmission*, 126 (3), 327–37 (<https://link.springer.com/article/10.1007/s00702-018-01967-w>, open-access).

The report of early-onset dementia due to a PSEN mutation is F. Lou et al. (2017), 'Very early-onset sporadic Alzheimer's disease with a de novo mutation in the PSEN1 gene', *Neurobiology of Aging*, 53, 193.e1-93.e5. (Available from <https://www.sciencedirect.com/science/article/pii/S0197458016303396>, this is not currently open-access.)

The UK Human Tissue Authority's guide to brain donation is available at <https://www.hta.gov.uk/guidance-public/brain-donation>.

The study comparing UK funding for dementia and other illnesses, such as cancer, is R. Luengo-Fernandez, J. Leal, and A. Gray (2015), 'UK research spend in 2008 and 2012: comparing stroke, cancer, coronary heart disease and dementia', *British Medical*

Journal Open, 5 (4), e006648 (full text available at <https://bmjopen.bmj.com/content/5/4/e006648>).

Data on global populations in 1965 and 2015 are taken from the UN website *World Population Prospects 2017*, which includes an interactive data facility, available at <https://population.un.org/wpp/DataQuery/>.

Data on UK populations in 1965 and 2015 are taken from the UK Office for National Statistics (ONS) population estimates; see e.g. <https://www.ons.gov.uk/peoplepopulationandcommunity/populationandmigration/populationestimates/datasets/populationestimatesforukenglandandwalesscotlandandnorthern-nireland>.

Chapter 2: What causes dementia?

The amyloid hypothesis was set out by J. A. Hardy and G. A. Higgins (1992), 'Alzheimer's disease: the amyloid cascade hypothesis', *Science*, 256 (5054), 184–5. (This article is not open-access, though *Science* will show you the first page for free at <http://science.sciencemag.org/content/256/5054/184/>.)

Information about *Sea Hero Quest* can be found at <http://www.seaheroquest.com/>.

The *APP* gene was reported by D. Goldgaber et al. (1987), 'Characterization and chromosomal localization of a cDNA encoding brain amyloid of Alzheimer's disease', *Science*, 235 (4791), 877–80 <(https://science.sciencemag.org/content/235/4791/877>, not open-access).

On the vexed question of common medications and dementia risk, see e.g. issue 361 of the *British Medical Journal* (2018) which contains research by K. Richardson et al., 'Anticholinergic drugs and risk of dementia: case-control study' (open-access from <https://www.bmj.com/content/361/bmj.k1315>), together with an editorial and comments ('rapid responses'). The editorial (S. L. Gray and J. T. Hanlon, 'Anticholinergic drugs and dementia in older adults', <https://www.bmj.com/content/361/bmj.k1722>) is unfortunately not open-access.

The purification of amyloid-beta was reported by G. G. Glenner and C. W. Wong (1984), 'Alzheimer's disease: initial report of the purification and characterization of a novel cerebrovascular amyloid protein', *Biochemical and Biophysical Research Communications*, 120 (3), 885–90. (This report, available via

ScienceDirect at <https://www.sciencedirect.com/science/article/pii/S0006291X84801904>, is not open-access.)

The case study relating *APOE* and *PSEN1* mutations is J. F. Arboleda-Velasquez et al. (2019), 'Resistance to autosomal dominant Alzheimer's disease in an APOE3 Christchurch homozygote: a case report', *Nature Medicine*, 25 (11), 1680–3 (<https://www.nature.com/articles/s41591-019-0611-3>, not open-access).

The study reporting a role for TDP-43 in skeletal muscle is T. O. Vogler et al. (2018), 'TDP-43 and RNA form amyloid-like myo-granules in regenerating muscle', *Nature*, 563 (7732), 508–13 (<https://www.nature.com/articles/s41586-018-0665-2, not open-access).

Chapter 3: Beyond amyloid

The Huntington's gene therapy trial is F. A. Siebzehnrübl et al. (2018), 'Early postnatal behavioral, cellular, and molecular changes in models of Huntington disease are reversible by HDAC inhibition', *Proceedings of the National Academy of Sciences USA*, 115 (37), E8765–E74. (Open-access, <https://www.pnas.org/content/115/37/E8765>.)

On brain injury and amyloid levels, the study referred to is S. Magnoni and D. L. Brody (2010), 'New perspectives on amyloid-beta dynamics after acute brain injury: moving between experimental approaches and studies in the human brain', *Archives of Neurology*, 67 (9), 1068–73 (<https://jamanetwork.com/journals/jamaneurology/fullarticle/801086>, open-access).

The study of amyloid-beta levels in CSF, suggesting that they drop long before symptoms appear, is C. L. Sutphen et al. (2015), 'Longitudinal cerebrospinal fluid biomarker changes in preclinical Alzheimer disease during middle age', *JAMA Neurology*, 72 (9), 1029–42. (This can be read on PubMed, at <https://www.ncbi.nlm.nih.gov/pmc/articles/PMC4570860/>.)

'Flogging a dead horse': the quotations 'from the leading journal *Nature*' are from researcher Peter Davies, cited in A. Abbott and E. Dolgin (2015), 'Failed Alzheimer's trial does not kill leading theory of disease', *Nature*, 540, 15–16. The full piece can be found at <https://www.nature.com/news/failed-alzheimer-s-trial-does-not-kill-leading-theory-of-disease-1.21045>.

The new classification system for biomarkers is described in C. R. Jack et al. (2016), 'A/T/N: An unbiased descriptive classification scheme for Alzheimer disease biomarkers', *Neurology*, 87 (5), 539–47 (<https://n.neurology.org/content/neurology/87/5/539.full.pdf>, PDF, open-access). For more on arguments over definitions, see D. S. Knopman et al. (2019), 'A brief history of "Alzheimer disease": multiple meanings separated by a common name', *Neurology*, 92 (22), 1053–9 (<https://n.neurology.org/content/92/22/1053>, not open-access).

The guidelines for vascular cognitive impairment are: O. A. Skrobot et al. (2016), 'Vascular cognitive impairment neuropathology guidelines (VCING): the contribution of cerebrovascular pathology to cognitive impairment', *Brain*, 139 (11), 2957–69 (<https://academic.oup.com/brain/article/139/11/2957/2422120>, open-access).

The disease LATE is described in P. T. Nelson et al. (2019), 'Limbic-predominant age-related TDP-43 encephalopathy (LATE): consensus working group report', *Brain*, 142 (6), 1503–27 (<http://www.ncbi.nlm.nih.gov/pubmed/31039256>, open-access).

The discovery that neutrophils can move from skull to brain is reported in F. Herisson et al. (2018), 'Direct vascular channels connect skull bone marrow and the brain surface enabling myeloid cell migration', *Nature Neuroscience*, 21 (9), 1209–17 (<https://www.nature.com/articles/s41593-018-0213-2>, not open-access).

Chapter 4: Risk factors

For a review and discussion of changes in dementia rates, including both Western nations and Japan and Nigeria, see Y.-T. Wu et al. (2017), 'The changing prevalence and incidence of dementia over time—current evidence', *Nature Reviews Neurology*, 13 (6), 327–39 (<https://www.nature.com/articles/nrneurol.2017.63>, not open-access). For the Chinese data, see Z. Bo et al. (2019), 'The temporal trend and distribution characteristics in mortality of Alzheimer's disease and other forms of dementia in China: based on the National Mortality Surveillance System (NMS) from 2009 to 2015', *PLoS ONE*, 14 (1), e0210621 (<https://journals.plos.org/plosone/article?id=10.1371/journal.pone.0210621>, open-access).

The large study of neurological disease risks is S. Licher et al. (2018), 'Lifetime risk of common neurological diseases in the elderly population', *Journal of Neurology, Neurosurgery and Psychiatry*, 90 (2), 148–56 (<https://jnnp.bmj.com/content/90/2/148>, open-access).

Nichols, E., et al. (2019), 'Global, regional, and national burden of Alzheimer's disease and other dementias, 1990–2016: a systematic analysis for the Global Burden of Disease Study 2016', *Lancet Neurology*, 18 (1), 88–106 (<https://www.thelancet.com/journals/laneur/article/PIIS1474-4422(18)30403-4/fulltext>, open-access).

The estimates of dementia prevalence in the UK are taken from table 1 of M. Prince et al. (2014), *Dementia UK* (second edition), King's College London/London School of Economics: for the Alzheimer's Society. The report is available at <https://www.alzheimers.org.uk/about-us/policy-and-influencing/dementia-uk-report?documentID=2759>.

For the WHO statistics and the estimates from Alzheimer Disease International, see the references for Chapter 1.

The study finding a more pronounced effect of air pollution on cognition in older people is X. Zhang et al. (2018), 'The impact of exposure to air pollution on cognitive performance', *Proceedings of the National Academy of Sciences USA*, 115 (37), 9193–7 (<http://www.pnas.org/content/115/37/9193>, open-access).

The 2014 American Heart Association/American Stroke Association statement, 'Factors influencing the decline in stroke mortality', is available from PubMed, at <https://www.ncbi.nlm.nih.gov/pmc/articles/PMC5995123/>.

For an optimistic review of the prospects for brain rejuvenation by parabiosis and other systemic (i.e. body-wide) methods, see J. Bouchard and S. A. Villeda (2015), 'Aging and brain rejuvenation as systemic events', *Journal of Neurochemistry*, 132 (1), 5–19. (This is open-access, available at <https://onlinelibrary.wiley.com/doi/full/10.1111/jnc.12969>.)

The meta-analysis on anti-cytokine treatments in depression is N. Kappelmann et al. (2016), 'Antidepressant activity of anti-cytokine treatment: a systematic review and meta-analysis of clinical trials of chronic inflammatory conditions', *Molecular Psychiatry*, 23 (2), 335–43. (This article, at <https://www.nature.com/articles/mp2016167>, is open-access.)

For more on regional variations in dementia, see e.g. R. N. Kalaria et al. (2008), 'Alzheimer's disease and vascular dementia in developing countries: prevalence, management, and risk factors', *Lancet Neurology*, 7 (9), 812–26 (available via PubMed at <https://www.

ncbi.nlm.nih.gov/pmc/articles/PMC2860610/>); V. Singh et al. (2018), 'Stroke risk and vascular dementia in South Asians', *Current Atherosclerosis Reports*, 20 (9), 43 (<https://link.springer. com/article/10.1007%2Fs11883-018-0745-7>, not open-access); W. B. Grant (2016), 'Using multicountry ecological and observational studies to determine dietary risk factors for Alzheimer's Disease', *Journal of the American College of Nutrition*, 35 (5), 476–89 (<https://www.tandfonline.com/doi/abs/10.1080/07315724.2016.1 161566>, not open-access); and S. Alladi and V. Hachinski (2018), 'World dementia: one approach does not fit all', *Neurology*, 91 (6), 264–70 (<https://n.neurology.org/content/91/6/264.long>, not open-access).

Chapter 5: Diagnosis and treatment

The two pieces featuring James E. Galvin as an author are J. E. Galvin and C. H. Sadowsky (2012), 'Practical guidelines for the recognition and diagnosis of dementia', *Journal of the American Board of Family Medicine*, 25 (3), 367–82 (available from <http://www. jabfm.org/content/25/3/367.abstract>); and J. E. Galvin (2017), 'Prevention of Alzheimer's disease: lessons learned and applied', *Journal of the American Geriatric Society*, 65 (10), 2128–33 (<https://onlinelibrary.wiley.com/doi/full/10.1111/jgs.14997>). Both are free to access.

The study of whether commonly used diagnostic tests for dementia are accurate is J. M. Ranson et al. (2019), 'Predictors of dementia misclassification when using brief cognitive assessments', *Neurology: Clinical Practice*, 9 (2), 109–17 (open-access, from <https://cp.neurology.org/content/9/2/109>).

Details of neurocognitive disorders are taken from the *DSM*'s current (2013) revision: *Diagnostic and Statistical Manual of Mental Disorders: DSM-5* (Washington, DC: American Psychiatric Publishing).

In the discussion of hospital care for people with dementia, the two studies mentioned are Ahsan Rao et al. (2016), 'Outcomes of dementia: systematic review and meta-analysis of hospital administrative database studies', *Archives of Gerontology and Geriatrics*, 66, 198–204; and S. Timmons et al. (2016), 'Acute hospital dementia care: results from a national audit', *BMC Geriatrics*, 16, 113. The Rao work is not freely available from the publisher (see <https://www.sciencedirect.com/science/article/

abs/pii/S0167494316301091>), but is available from the authors'
institution (<https://spiral.imperial.ac.uk:8443/handle/
10044/1/38730>) as a Microsoft Word document. The work by
Timmons and colleagues is open-access (<https://bmcgeriatr.
biomedcentral.com/articles/10.1186/s12877-016-0293-3>).

The Royal College of Psychiatrists' *National Audit of Dementia Care in
General Hospitals 2016–2017* is available online from the
Healthcare Quality Improvement Partnership, an independent
organization, at <https://www.hqip.org.uk/wp-content/
uploads/2018/02/national-audit-of-dementia-care-in-general-
hospitals-2016-2017-third-round-of-audit-report.pdf>.

A guide to the searchable ClinicalTrials.gov database, run by the US
National Institutes for Health (NIH) but incorporating trials from
around the world, is available at <https://www.clinicaltrials.gov/>.

An EU-based source for the estimates of clinical trial non-reporting
can be found at <https://eu.trialstracker.net/>.

The review of non-pharmacological interventions (NPIs) by Ann
Kolanowski and colleagues is A. Kolanowski et al. (2018),
'Advancing research on care needs and supportive approaches for
persons with dementia: recommendations and rationale', *JAMDA*
(the *Journal of the American Medical Directors Association*), 19
(12), 1047–53. (The abstract is available at <https://www.jamda.
com/article/S1525-8610(18)30387-6/abstract>, but the full text is
not freely available.)

A guide to Cochrane reviews can be found at <https://www.
cochranelibrary.com/about/about-cochrane-reviews>.

On Montessori methods, see C. L. Sheppard et al. (2016) 'A systematic
review of Montessori-based activities for persons with dementia',
JAMDA, 17 (2), 117–22 (the abstract is provided at <https://www.
jamda.com/article/S1525-8610(15)00643-X/fulltext>, but the
review itself is not currently open-access).

Jütten, L. H., et al. (2018), 'The effectiveness of psychosocial and
behavioral interventions for informal dementia caregivers:
meta-analyses and meta-regressions', *Journal of Alzheimer's and
Dementia*, 66 (1), 149–72 (<https://content.iospress.com/articles/
journal-of-alzheimers-disease/jad180508>, not open-access).

The 2010 review giving five principles for NPIs is H. Yamaguchi et al.
(2010), 'Overview of non-pharmacological intervention for
dementia and principles of brain-activating rehabilitation',
Psychogeriatrics, 10 (4), 206–13 (<https://onlinelibrary.wiley.com/
doi/full/10.1111/j.1479-8301.2010.00323.x>, open-access).

Chapter 6: The future of dementia

The Alzheimer's Society and Alzheimer's Association estimates of dementia carers' economic contributions in the UK and USA are given on their respective websites: 'Key Facts' (<https://www.alzheimers.org.uk/about-us/news-and-media/facts-media>) and 'Facts and Figures' (<https://alz.org/alzheimers-dementia/facts-figures>). The estimate for Japan is from M. Sado et al. (2018), 'The estimated cost of dementia in Japan, the most aged society in the world', *PLoS ONE*, 13 (11), e0206508 (open-access at <https://journals.plos.org/plosone/article?id=10.1371/journal.pone.0206508>).

The report on global economic costs of dementia care by Alzheimer's Disease International is available from their website, <https://www.alz.co.uk/news/global-estimates-of-informal-care>.

The 2018 UK government spending figures are from <https://www.ukpublicspending.co.uk/>.

Further reading

For a readable and wide-ranging overview of the state of dementia research, see K. Taylor (2016), *The Fragile Brain: The Strange, Hopeful Science of Dementia* (Oxford: Oxford University Press).

A useful guide to specific neurodegenerative disorders can be found at the website of the US National Institute of Neurological Disorders and Stroke, <https://www.ninds.nih.gov/>. It covers the common conditions and many rare ones. For more about rarer forms of dementia, see the <http://www.raredementiasupport.org/> website, run by the Dementia Research Centre at University College London, which offers support for frontotemporal dementia, posterior cortical atrophy, primary progressive aphasia, and familial Alzheimer's; or for dementia with Lewy bodies, see the Lewy Body Society, <https://www.lewybody.org/>.

Information about the latest dementia research, as well as practical guidance to managing the various types of dementia, is plentiful online. See the 'Useful organizations and websites' section for sources.

For a review, and defence, of the (updated) amyloid cascade hypothesis of dementia, see D. J. Selkoe and J. Hardy (2016), 'The amyloid hypothesis of Alzheimer's disease at 25 years', *EMBO Molecular Medicine*, 8 (6), 595–608 (free to read at <http://www.ncbi.nlm.nih.gov/pmc/articles/PMC4888851/>).

For a critique of the amyloid cascade hypothesis, and discussion of alternatives, see K. Herrup (2015), 'The case for rejecting the amyloid cascade hypothesis', *Nature Neuroscience*, 794–9 (<https://www.nature.com/articles/nn.4017>, not open-access).

For more details on the role of inflammatory immune processes in the brain, see M. T. Heneka et al. (2015), 'Innate immunity in

Alzheimer's disease', *Nature Immunology* 16 (3), 229–36 (<https://www.nature.com/articles/ni.3102>, not open-access).

For further reading on the preventable risks of dementia, and lifestyle changes that may help, see G. Livingston et al. (2017), 'Dementia prevention, intervention, and care', *Lancet*, 390 (10113), 2673–734 (<https://www.thelancet.com/journals/lancet/article/PIIS0140-6736(17)31363-6/fulltext>, free with registration); N. Mukadam et al. (2019), 'Population attributable fractions for risk factors for dementia in low-income and middle-income countries: an analysis using cross-sectional survey data', *Lancet Global Health*, 7 (5), e596-e603 (<https://www.thelancet.com/journals/langlo/article/PIIS2214-109X(19)30074-9/fulltext>, open-access); and M. Kivipelto et al. (2018), 'Lifestyle interventions to prevent cognitive impairment, dementia and Alzheimer disease', *Nature Reviews Neurology*, 14 (11), 653–66 (<https://www.nature.com/articles/s41582-018-0070-3>, not open-access).

For a scientifically informed overview of the implications for policy of the rapidly ageing population, in this case in the UK, see the government's 2016 Foresight Report, *Future of an Ageing Population*, available from: <https://www.gov.uk/government/publications/future-of-an-ageing-population>.

When considering dementia care, many commentators remark that the biomedical model which dominates research is less helpful than a more person-centred approach. One of the most influential exponents of this way of thinking was undoubtedly Professor Thomas (Tom) Kitwood, who among much else developed the methods of dementia care mapping to make formal care institutions more person-centred. His ideas are clearly set out in his book *Dementia Reconsidered: The Person Comes First* (McGraw-Hill Education, 1997). More information about dementia care mapping is available from Bradford University: <https://www.bradford.ac.uk/dementia/dementia-care-mapping/>.

For a perspective from someone living with dementia, try <https://kateswaffer.com/>. For a guide to how different societies are approaching the question of how best to help people with dementia live well, there is Camilla Cavendish's book *Extra Time: 10 Lessons for an Ageing World* (HarperCollins, 2019). For a thoughtful guide to reimagining dementia in terms of disability and human rights, see Suzanne Cahill's book *Dementia and Human Rights* (Policy Press, 2018).

Useful organizations and websites

Please note that listings in this section are provided for information and do not represent endorsements of the organizations. Hyperlinks are correct as of March 2020.

Governments and international organizations

UK Care Quality Commission (independent regulator)
<https://www.cqc.org.uk/help-advice>

UK National Health Service (NHS)
Information about diagnosis: <https://www.nhs.uk/conditions/dementia/diagnosis/>.
Help available: <https://www.nhs.uk/conditions/dementia/social-services-and-the-nhs/>.

UK National Institute for Clinical Excellence (NICE) guidelines
<https://www.nice.org.uk/guidance/ng97/chapter/recommendations>.

US American Psychological Association (APA)
Information about dementia: <http://www.apa.org/helpcenter/living-with-dementia.aspx>.
Guidelines for practitioners: <http://www.apa.org/practice/guidelines/dementia.aspx>.
Comparison of *ICD* and *DSM*: <http://www.apa.org/monitor/2009/10/icd-dsm.aspx>.

US National Institute on Aging (NIA)
<https://www.nia.nih.gov/health/alzheimers>.

US National Institute of Neurological Disorders and Stroke
.

World Health Organization (WHO)
Information about the *ICD*: <http://www.who.int/classifications/icd/en/>.
Information about dementia: <http://www.who.int/mental_health/neurology/dementia/en/>.

Charities and dementia societies

Alzheimer Europe
<https://www.alzheimer-europe.org/>.

Alzheimer Society of Canada
Homepage: <https://alzheimer.ca/en/Home>.
Charter of Rights for People with Dementia: <https://alzheimer.ca/en/Home/Get-involved/ The-Charter>.

Alzheimer's Association (US)
<https://www.alz.org/>.

Alzheimer's Disease International (a federation of dementia societies)
Homepage: <https://www.alz.co.uk/>.
World Alzheimer Report 2018: <https://www.alz.co.uk/research/world-report-2018>.

Alzheimer's Society (UK)
<https://www.alzheimers.org.uk/>.

Carers Trust (UK)
<https://carers.org/key-facts-about-carers-and-people-they-care>.

Dementia UK
<https://www.dementiauk.org/>.

Help Age International
<http://www.helpage.org/>.

YoungDementiaUK
<https://www.youngdementiauk.org/>.

Research trials
The USA and EU maintain public registries of clinical trials for many
conditions. More information about these can be found at: <www.
ClinicalTrials.gov> and <www.clinicaltrialsregister.eu>. For
dementia research trials, more information can be found at:

Alzheimer Europe
<https://www.alzheimer-europe.org/Research/Clinical-Trials-Watch>.

Alzheimer's Association
<https://www.alz.org/alzheimers-dementia/research_progress/
clinical-trials>.

Alzheimer's Research UK
<https://www.alzheimersresearchuk.org/about-dementia/
helpful-information/getting-involved-in-research/>.

AlzForum therapeutics database
<https://www.alzforum.org/therapeutics>.

Join Dementia Research (UK)
<https://www.joindementiaresearch.nihr.ac.uk/>.

Specific treatment methods

Cochrane reviews (searchable database)
<https://www.cochranelibrary.com/cdsr/reviews>.

Cognitive stimulation therapy
<http://www.cstdementia.com/>.

Montessori method
<https://www.mariamontessori.org/training/what-we-offer/
dementia/>.

Publisher's acknowledgements

We are grateful for permission to include the following copyright material in this book.

Extract reproduced with permission from K. Maurer, S. Volk, and H. Gerbaldo, 'Auguste D and Alzheimer's disease', *Lancet*, 349 (9064), 1546–9.

Index

For the benefit of digital users, indexed terms that span two pages (e.g., 52–53) may, on occasion, appear on only one of those pages.

SLEEP
A Very Short Introduction
Russell G. Foster & Steven W. Lockley

Why do we need sleep? What happens when we don't get enough? From the biology and psychology of sleep and the history of sleep in science, art, and literature; to the impact of a 24/7 society and the role of society in causing sleep disruption, this *Very Short Introduction* addresses the biological and psychological aspects of sleep, providing a basic understanding of what sleep is and how it is measured, looking at sleep through the human lifespan and the causes and consequences of major sleep disorders. Russell G. Foster and Steven W. Lockley go on to consider the impact of modern society, examining the relationship between sleep and work hours, and the impact of our modern lifestyle.

MEMORY
A Very Short Introduction
Michael J. Benton

Why do we remember events from our childhood as if they happened yesterday, but not what we did last week? Why does our memory seem to work well sometimes and not others? What happens when it goes wrong? Can memory be improved or manipulated, by psychological techniques or even 'brain implants'? How does memory grow and change as we age? And what of so-called 'recovered' memories? This book brings together the latest research in neuroscience and psychology, and weaves in case-studies, anecdotes, and even literature and philosophy, to address these and many other important questions about the science of memory - how it works, and why we can't live without it.

www.oup.com/vsi

HIV/AIDS
A Very Short Introduction
Alan Whiteside

HIV/AIDS is without doubt the worst epidemic to hit humankind since the Black Death. The first case was identified in 1981; by 2004 it was estimated that about 40 million people were living with the disease, and about 20 million had died. The news is not all bleak though. There have been unprecedented breakthroughs in understanding diseases and developing drugs. Because the disease is so closely linked to sexual activity and drug use, the need to understand and change behaviour has caused us to reassess what it means to be human and how we should operate in the globalising world. This *Very Short Introduction* provides an introduction to the disease, tackling the science, the international and local politics, the fascinating demographics, and the devastating consequences of the disease, and explores how we have — and must — respond.

'It won't make you an expert. But you'll know what you're talking about and you'll have a better idea of all the work we still have to do to wrestle this monster to the ground.'

Aids-free world website.

GENIUS
A Very Short Introduction
Andrew Robinson

Genius is highly individual and unique, of course, yet it shares a compelling, inevitable quality for professionals and the general public alike. Darwin's ideas are still required reading for every working biologist; they continue to generate fresh thinking and experiments around the world. So do Einstein's theories among physicists. Shakespeare's plays and Mozart's melodies and harmonies continue to move people in languages and cultures far removed from their native England and Austria. Contemporary 'geniuses' may come and go, but the idea of genius will not let go of us. Genius is the name we give to a quality of work that transcends fashion, celebrity, fame, and reputation: the opposite of a period piece. Somehow, genius abolishes both the time and the place of its origin.

EPIDEMIOLOGY
A Very Short Introduction
Rodolfo Saracci

Epidemiology has had an impact on many areas of medicine; and lung cancer, to the origin and spread of new epidemics. and lung cancer, to the origin and spread of new epidemics. However, it is often poorly understood, largely due to misrepresentations in the media. In this *Very Short Introduction* Rodolfo Saracci dispels some of the myths surrounding the study of epidemiology. He provides a general explanation of the principles behind clinical trials, and explains the nature of basic statistics concerning disease. He also looks at the ethical and political issues related to obtaining and using information concerning patients, and trials involving placebos.

WITCHCRAFT
A Very Short Introduction
Malcolm Gaskill

Witchcraft is a subject that fascinates us all, and everyone knows what a witch is - or do they? From childhood most of us develop a sense of the mysterious, malign person, usually an old woman. Historically, too, we recognize witch-hunting as a feature of modern societies. But why do witches still feature so heavily in cultures and consciousness? From Halloween to superstition and literary references such as Faust and even Harry Potter, witches still feature heavily in our society. In this Very Short Introduction Malcolm Gaskill challenges all of this, and argues that what we think we know is, in fact, wrong.

> 'Each chapter in this small but perfectly-formed book could be the jumping-off point for a year's stimulating reading. Buy it now.'
>
> Fortean Times